THE **Snoring Cure**

SIMPLE STEPS

TO GETTING

A GOOD NIGHT'S SLEEP

W. W. Norton & Company

NEW YORK • LONDON

Copyright © 1999 by Laurence A. Smolley, M.D., and
Debra Fulghum Bruce

For information about permission to reproduce selections from this
book, write to Permissions, W. W. Norton & Company, Inc., 500
Fifth Avenue, New York, NY 10110

The text of this book is composed in Bembo with the display set
in Modula
Composition by JoAnn Schambier
Manufacturing by the Maple-Vail Book Manufacturing Group
Book design by Judith Stagnitto Abbate/Abbate Design

Library of Congress Cataloging-in-Publication Data

Smolley, Laurence A.
    The snoring cure : simple steps to getting a good night's
    sleep / Laurence A. Smolley and Debra Fulghum Bruce.
        p.   cm.
    Includes index.
    ISBN 0-393-04742-3
    1. Snoring—Popular works. I. Bruce, Debra Fulghum, 1951–
II. Title.
    RA786.3 .S66 1999
    616.8'498—dc21
                                                        98-50594
                                                             CIP

W. W. Norton & Company, Inc., 500 Fifth Avenue, New York,
N.Y. 10110
www.wwnorton.com

W. W. Norton & Company Ltd., 10 Coptic Street, London
WC1A 1PU

1 2 3 4 5 6 7 8 9 0

THE Snoring Cure

Laurence A. Smolley, M.D.

A N D

Debra Fulghum Bruce

TO OUR FAMILIES:
DANI, NOAM, SARA, ARON, BEN, AND MARTHA SMOLLEY;
ROB, CLAIRE, BRITT, ASHLEY, AND BOB BRUCE

CONTENTS

ACKNOWLEDGMENTS

We have received generous assistance, along with a wealth of up-to-date information, from a very select group of health care professionals. We express our gratitude to the following from the Cleveland Clinic Florida, Fort Lauderdale:

Kendall Hanft, M.D., and Frank Astor, M.D., Department of Otolaryngology, for the chapter on surgical treatments of obstructive sleep apnea.

Jeffrey Wolkowicz, M.D., Chairman, Department of Pulmonary Diseases, for sections on the medical complications of obstructive sleep apnea.

Selim Benbadis, M.D., Department of Neurology and co-medical director of the Sleep Disorders Center, for sections on excessive daytime sleepiness.

We are also grateful to

Marcel Deray, M.D., Department of Neurology, Miami Childrens Hospital, Miami, Florida, for the sections on sleep apnea in children.

Irys Caristo, Department of Pulmonary Disease, Cleveland Clinic Florida, Fort Lauderdale. Without her excellent secretarial skills, the processing of much of this text would not have been possible.

Samuel Benjamin Smolley, who helped make our communication through cyberspace possible. Without him, we would still be depending on snail mail!

Brittnye and Ashley Bruce, whose research into weight loss and sleep problems gave new insight for those who need to lose weight to cure snoring.

THE Snoring Cure

S.O.S.– Stop Our Snoring

I f you've ever dreamed of sleeping through the night without snoring; if you live from sunrise to sundown on coffee, tea, and caffeinated drinks just to function minimally; if you fall asleep easily when you sit to watch television during the day; or if your bed partner has moved to the other end of the house, complaining that your nightly thunderous snores might win you a spot in the *Guinness Book of World Records*; then *this book will help*! We want to start you on the road to sounder sleep, increased energy and productivity, and better health as you stop snoring . . . forever.

Snoring is a universal complaint that affects more than 40 million men and women (and their bed partners, family members, and coworkers). Realizing the impact of this medical problem on millions, we wrote this book to give new hope to those who snore night after night. It will educate you about snoring and how it can literally "rob you of life," as it is associated with such serious problems as daytime sleepiness, memory loss, depression, hypertension, cardiovascular disease, and stroke.

This book will teach you how to stop snoring at a rate of almost *100 percent*. If you snore, if you sleep with a snorer, or if you work with a snorer, especially one who cannot concentrate on work because of daytime fatigue, this book promises to change your life.

MORE THAN NOISE

Interestingly, when the first book on sleep disorders was published in 1968, only 22 pages were devoted to snoring. Until that time, most scientists assumed that snoring was simply an annoying nuisance. There were no studies or hints that snoring was associated with heart disease, stroke, or even death at that time.

Today we know differently. In the early 1970s, epidemiological studies began to reveal startling evidence that snoring was *far greater* than a noisy distraction. Through a host of scientific studies, it became clear that some serious health problems are much more frequent among habitual snorers. Snoring may indeed be a warning symptom or red flag for a more serious problem called *obstructive sleep apnea* (OSA), a condition in which the airway behind the tongue is blocked off intermittently during sleep. (The abbreviation "OSA" will frequently be used through this book.)

So much myth and lack of information surround snoring that many people are shocked to find out that snoring is correlated with the extra girth accumulated through the years. It is also associated with high blood pressure. With the new surge of information on impotence, millions of men who suffer with erectile dysfunction are astounded when the urologist links their impotency with something as seemingly benign as nighttime snoring.

Did you know that waking up during the night to go to the bathroom is also correlated with snoring? One forty-five-year-old man who awakened frequently to urinate was convinced he had prostate disease until a sleep study confirmed snoring associated with OSA. Another middle-aged woman who suffered with congestion could not believe that her breathing disorders caused her continual snoring and subsequent daytime sleepiness. She was so tired at work that she could no longer think clearly, remember names, or even concentrate—until she began treatment for her nasal congestion and stopped snoring. Do you see why a cure for snoring may change your life forever?

NOT A LAUGHING MATTER

If you snore, it is time to come out of your hiding place. The jokes are over, and we take this problem seriously. Perhaps this is the first book ever written that does *not* blame you for snoring, but gives you workable tools for understanding this medical problem and taking action to stop it. After all, do you want to be haunted your entire lifetime by this irritating, roaring sound that flows out of your throat during sleep? Of course not! Does your bed partner relish staying awake night after night, poking you in the side in hopes that you will quit? We doubt it! Or, has your partner already moved to another room at the other end of your home to avoid being awakened? Probably! This will all change when you start the **4-step cure** in this book.

NEW HOPE FOR AN AGING POPULATION

If you are over age 35, you know that staying young, feeling energetic, and being productive are the quintessential goals to compete in today's marketplace. No, we cannot change the inevitable; we all will grow old. However, we can stop problems that are often associated with aging such as snoring, which can rob you of precious sleep, vitality, youthfulness, . . . and your health.

As the title of this book indicates, *this 4-step program really does work*! But—we cannot forget to mention—once you are cured of snoring, the chances are great that you will also receive important health-extending benefits such as

- **Heightened immune function.** Snoring is likely to disrupt your sleep cycle, resulting in less REM (rapid eye movement) sleep as discussed on pages 7–10. It is during the deepest level of sleep that the body is revitalized and tissue damage repaired. In fact, lack of deep sleep is associated with reduced immune function. Taking care of the snoring will enable you to sleep more soundly through the night, greatly enhancing your body's ability to resist disease and infections.

- **Reduced blood pressure.** More than one-third of those with hypertension also have OSA. The majority of those with severe sleep apnea are hypertensive. Uncontrolled hypertension can lead to serious cardiovascular problems, including increased risk of angina and heart disease. Fortunately, hypertension often improves after treatment of OSA.

- **Improved cardiovascular functioning.** If you snore and also have OSA, chances are your cardiovascular system is being greatly stressed. Studies show that habitual snorers have a greater chance of stroke than nonsnorers have. It is not unusual for those with sleep apnea to be mistakenly treated for primary heart disease because abnormal heart rhythms may be *more* prominent than the breathing disturbances. When breathing stops during the apneas, your heart rate changes. It may become very fast, very slow, or very irregular. This may result in less blood being pumped out and an increase in blood pressure. When breathing resumes, your heart rate and blood pressure rise, sometimes to very dangerous levels. These problems are lessened when treatment begins to correct the snoring and OSA.

- **Increased sex drive.** It has long been suspected that hypertension and penile erectile dysfunction or impotence are associated with each other. Some medications for hypertension and other medical problems can also cause male sexual dysfunction. Because impotence is directly related to snoring in men with OSA, taking care of this may often help solve associated sexual problems, including erectile dysfunction. For the "pure" snorer (or snoring not associated with OSA), simply ending the snoring will allow your bed partner to move back into your bed and sleep with you once again. That in itself may solve many sexual problems!

- **Greater energy, alertness, and productivity.** Sleep deprivation caused by snoring can make you feel moody, tired, and mentally impaired. In fact, researchers claim that those who snore have more car accidents and sick days than nonsnorers have. People who snore also have poor concentration and impaired memory, and do poorly on psychological testing. This may be caused by the low levels of oxygen in their blood and by the fragmented sleep. Yet correcting the problem may let you experience a higher quality of continuous sleep and rejuvenate your body.

Based upon scientifically sound studies, this book will educate you about important factors that contribute to snoring, fitful sleep, and the resulting health problems, and then will show you how unhealthy lifestyle habits such as overeating, nighttime eating, heavy alcohol consumption, and cigarette smoking can worsen the problem. The **4-step cure** will also give you practical and easy-to-implement tools to make important lifestyle changes, controlling those risk factors you can change, and guide you toward appropriate medical therapy or surgical treatments, if warranted.

Enough about what this book will do to improve your health and your life. Let's now get started, for it is our utmost hope that upon trying the 4-step cure, you and your loved ones *snore no more!*

CHAPTER 1

Good Sleep, Bad Sleep...No Sleep

Y ou never think about sleep . . . until you awaken feeling exhausted. If you snore, you probably wish you could have *good sleep*, yet most snorers experience *bad or restless sleep*. Sadly, their bed partners or family members may tell of having *no sleep*.

"Why is sleep so important anyway? I can get by on four hours of sleep during busy weeks." Rachel's narrow assessment of her need for sleep is probably a big reason why her social life is on the decline! After all, lack of sleep makes you feel tired and irritable all day long. Remember going to those all-night slumber parties in high school? Or, did you ever pull an "all-nighter" in college during exam week? Think about how you felt the next day. Most people would admit to feeling oversensitive, light-headed, fatigued, and lethargic.

"But I just can't sleep. I try to relax, but my mind is filled with all the commitments I have for the next day. After tossing and turning for several hours, I get angry and finally just give up and work on my computer. I am so sleepy the next day that I can hardly function." Pete's sleep problem is nothing new to millions of adults. Nearly one in three people surveyed by the National Sleep

Foundation reported getting *only six hours or less of sleep during the week*—although 98 percent of those surveyed said sleep was as important to them as exercise and good nutrition.

So, what's wrong with lack of sleep? Plenty, say experts. Of those, like Pete, who tell of having daytime sleepiness, nearly 37 percent say lack of sleep affects their normal activities. This results in a 30 percent reduction in job performance, and performance of family duties falls by 50 percent. The cost of sleep problems, including snoring and obstructive sleep apnea, to the nation exceeds $15.9 billion in direct costs (see Table 1.1), as well as $50 to $100 billion in indirect yet related costs, such as accidents and court costs.

Sleep deprivation is a stress that definitely has significant physiological consequences (high blood pressure or heart complications), as well as psychological consequences (see Table 1.2), that result in serious and sometimes deadly problems. As many as 23 percent of Americans have actually fallen asleep while driving, and according to the National Highway Traffic Safety Administration, at least 100,000 crashes and 1,500 deaths occur annually as a result of drowsy drivers. Industrial accidents can also occur, such as the terrible oil spill of the Exxon *Valdez* that happened because the first mate was asleep at the wheel and ignored warning signals.

TABLE 1.1	

The Direct Costs of Poor Sleep and Mental Impairment

Reduced productivity
Increased incidence of motor-vehicle accidents
Increased incidence of coronary artery disease and heart attacks
Increased incidence of industrial accidents
Increased incidence of accidental injuries and deaths at work
Increased incidence of medical and psychiatric illnesses
Increased incidence of employee turnover and retraining

TABLE 1.2	

Psychological Consequences of Sleep Deprivation

Mood swings
Irritability
Depression
Lack of patience
Intolerance
Problems with brain function
Forgetfulness
Difficulty learning
Decreased attention span
Negligence
Reduced performance

THE REAL PROBLEM WITH LACK OF SLEEP

The most serious problem of poor sleep is that it affects every part of your life, from your relationships, to your ability to think and be creative, to your income. After all, it's difficult to make a living if you are not alert or productive on the job.

To help you understand how sleep affects you personally, let's first analyze the intimate connection between sleep and breathing—two extremely important functions that most of us take for granted. Think about it. If you stopped breathing, death would follow within minutes, as your brain would starve for life-sustaining oxygen. However, not many consider the deleterious outcomes of lack of sleep.

OXYGEN IN, CARBON DIOXIDE OUT

Normal breathing is necessary for getting oxygen into the body and carbon dioxide out of the body. You can thank your *respiratory system*

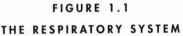

FIGURE 1.1
THE RESPIRATORY SYSTEM

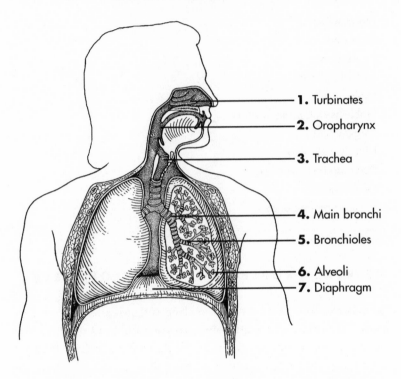

1. Turbinates

2. Oropharynx

3. Trachea

4. Main bronchi

5. Bronchioles

6. Alveoli
7. Diaphragm

(see Figure 1.1) for this function. Your lungs are the main part of the respiratory system. Yet your nose, throat, trachea or main windpipe, chest wall, and certain muscles, such as the diaphragm, are all part of your respiratory system and play important roles in breathing.

The main goal of your respiratory system is to keep the blood levels of oxygen, carbon dioxide, and acid normal so the cells in your body can function properly. Therefore, if your oxygen levels fall or carbon dioxide levels rise, your rate of breathing will increase at an appropriate pace on demand.

While you are asleep, your body's response to these low levels of oxygen or high levels of carbon dioxide may be inadequate, making it difficult to maintain normal levels. Difficulty maintaining near-normal levels of the blood gases and the acid balance in the bloodstream may be more pronounced if you have a lung problem such as asthma, chronic bronchitis, or emphysema.

THE BODY'S GATEKEEPER

While many people think the respiratory system starts in the airways closest to the lungs, it actually begins in your nose. Besides helping you smell your environment, the main function of your nose is as a "gatekeeper," protecting the lower airways from dry, cold, or contaminated air. When you breathe in, this air temperature is adjusted close to body temperature as it travels through the nose. At the same time, air is moisturized, and particles in the air are filtered out.

You may secretly wish the outward appearance of your nose were smaller or more perky; however, the insides of everyone's noses function in very much the same way. The openings of your nose, or *nostrils*, are lined with skin and a thin mesh of hair, which projects into the airway to provide the first filter for dust or other particles such as pollen, smoke, or bacteria.

Even though you cannot see what is happening inside the nose, you may have noticed your nose becoming clogged, especially when you lie on your back or your side. Since your nasal passages are not very wide, it doesn't take much to cause obstruction. Part of the reason why obstruction occurs when you lie down is that tissue fluids and blood pool in the head, causing swelling and possibly blockage in the nasal passages. Occasionally, both sides of your nasal passages become blocked, causing you to breathe through your mouth. This may account for your dry mouth when you awaken in the morning. Mouth breathing is more likely to be associated with snoring.

NORMAL SLEEP: TIME AND STAGES

To help you understand how changes in resistance at the back of the throat during sleep can affect your quality of sleep, let's first look at what constitutes "normal" sleep. Normal adults usually sleep seven to eight hours each night. You may need more, or you may get by very well with less. There are those who may brag about needing fewer than four hours, but they are often simply fooling themselves.

No matter how much sleep you get, restful sleep—good sleep—is necessary to help heal and repair your body, especially as you age. Newborn babies need sixteen or seventeen hours of sleep each day, about eight hours during the night and about eight hours during daylight divided into many naps. As the child gets older, she will spend more time asleep at night and less time napping during the day. By age four, the preschool child is sleeping about ten to twelve hours per night without any naps. Then, with age, there is a gradual decrease in nighttime sleep down to the normal adult amount.

Comprehensive scientific studies now suggest that a complex of nerve cells and interconnections within the brain is responsible for the cycles of sleep and wakefulness. You have a built-in cycle of sleep-wake times called *circadian rhythms* (*circa* means "around," and *dia* means "day"). These cycles are controlled by a group of nerve cells called a *circadian pacemaker*, which is closely related to parts of the retina in the back of your eyes and the hypothalamus in your brain. The hypothalamus controls many functions of the body throughout the day.

The circadian cycle is actually twenty-five hours long. Since this cycle is longer than the twenty-four-hour day, there must be some coordination between the body's pacemaker and the external clock time. Such coordination is controlled by cues in the environment, and the most powerful one is *light*.

Under normal circumstances, you awaken in the morning in response to some cue such as an alarm clock or sunlight beaming through your bedroom window. As the morning hours advance, you get more alert until about 1:00 P.M. or 2:00 P.M., when you have a lull or sag in wakefulness. Although you may think this dip in alertness was caused by the heaping platter of lasagna you ate at lunchtime, this is not so. The lull is a natural consequence of your circadian rhythm. Interestingly, some cultures such as those in Latin America and in the Middle East incorporate this lull into each day's schedule by taking a siesta (or nap) in the early afternoon, then getting back to work later on. Later in the afternoon, you become more alert and energetic again until late evening when you start to experience a wave of sleepiness. With your usual bedtime ritual, you will fall asleep until the next morning when the cycle starts again.

THE STAGES OF SLEEP

Even though there are varying differences with circadian rhythms and sleep styles, we all have one thing in common—we need good sleep to be energetic, to be alert, and to stay healthy. Sleep is made up of distinct stages with specific characteristics defined by brain waves, eye movements, and muscle tension. In a sleep lab, these stages are recorded by electroencephalography (EEG), electrooculography (EOG), and electromyography (EMG), as defined on page 54. The two broad categories of sleep include rapid eye movement (REM) sleep and nonrapid eye movement (NREM) sleep.

During REM sleep, there are small, variable-speed brain waves, rapid eye movements like those of eyes-open wakefulness, and no muscle tension. It is during REM sleep that you have most of your dreams. (When you are aroused from REM sleep, you may have recall of vivid imagery.) NREM sleep is composed of four different levels or stages—1, 2, 3, and 4—characterized by different combinations of brain waves, eye movements, and reduced but not absent muscle tension (see Table 1.3).

Your sleep intensity or quality is reflected by the amount of *delta sleep* you get each night. Delta sleep (stages 3 and 4) is the deepest level of sleep, a regenerative period during which your body heals itself. Growth hormone secretion is highest during

TABLE 1.3	

Stages of Sleep

Stage 1—light sleep
Stage 2—moderate sleep
Stages 3 and 4—deep or delta sleep
REM (rapid eye movement) sleep or dream stage

delta sleep, and some researchers believe that this is important for growth and repair of body tissue.

Delta sleep occurs mostly in the first third of the night and makes up about 10 to 20 percent of total nighttime sleep in normal young adults. REM sleep takes place mostly during the last third of your night's sleep and comprises normally 25 percent of the sleep period.

The percentage of delta sleep is affected by age, amount of prior sleep, and various diseases. As a rule, delta sleep decreases with age and may be brief in healthy, elderly males. If you do not get enough delta sleep, you will feel tired and groggy the next day.

Not surprisingly, young children have particularly large proportions of delta sleep, which increases if they are sleep deprived. This explains why trying to wake up a young child may be difficult. Elderly people have smaller proportions of delta sleep, which is why they can be easily aroused by environmental noise. Medical problems such as obstructive sleep apnea, periodic leg movements during sleep, or fibromyalgia (an arthritis-like syndrome) may affect both the quantity and the quality of delta sleep. This, in turn, probably accounts for the feeling of fatigue experienced by people suffering from these ailments. Other results of poor sleep are listed in Table 1.4.

NOW, SAY "AHHH" AND BREATHE

If you've ever watched someone breathe through the mouth during sleep, you know how odd it looks and how it may cause that

TABLE 1.4	

Results of Poor Sleep

Daytime fatigue

Increased aches and pains

Illness

Depression, irritability, and moodiness

Declining fitness and endurance

Reduced activity

Morning headache

person to crave water in the morning to quench the dryness. Yet mouth breathing is also a serious problem where sleep problems are concerned, causing problems from bad breath to sore throat to snoring.

While you sleep, your respiratory system continues to be hard at work. The muscles at the back of your throat tend to relax while your diaphragm continues its pumping action. The excessive relaxation of the muscles in the mouth, throat, and neck results in blockage of airflow. If this blockage is occasional, the soft palate and uvula (that fleshy and sometimes long and swollen structure that hangs down from your soft palate) in the back of the throat (see Figure 1.2) may shake, flop back and forth, or vibrate, causing the annoying noises we call *snoring*. If this obstruction is prolonged, a *cessation* or *pause of breathing* known as an *apnea* may happen. When apneas are long enough, there may be a drop in blood oxygen supplies, along with a host of other serious problems discussed in Chapter 3.

In NREM sleep, your breathing will be remarkably regular. Yet, there is a tendency for the speed of *inspiration* (breathing in) to be decreased as you go into progressively deeper stages of NREM sleep. There is also an increase in upper-airway resistance at the base of the tongue toward the back of the throat. This resistance occurs

FIGURE 1.2

COMMON ANATOMICAL FEATURES OF SNORERS

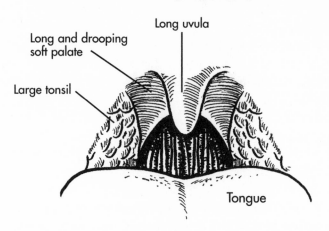

because of fewer nerve signals sent to muscles in that region of your body. When you are awake and active, these nerve signals keep the airway open.

Breathing during REM sleep is irregular, and you experience a sudden variability in both the size and the frequency of breaths. You may have apneas in which your breathing actually stops for 10 to 30 seconds. These sudden changes occur just when there are bursts of rapid eye movement. The contribution of the rib cage to breathing during REM sleep is decreased because of reduced activity of the muscle between your ribs. The muscles of the chest wall located in between the ribs become very relaxed during REM sleep. This causes the chest cavity to become smaller and the size of the lungs themselves to be smaller. For those with emphysema or bronchitis, smaller lung volumes may result in low oxygen levels.

Also, during REM sleep, diaphragm activity is increased, and the muscles that keep the upper airway open are almost complete-ly relaxed. As we discuss in Chapter 3, obstructive sleep apnea may be most severe during REM sleep because of this.

WHO'S AT RISK?

....

While most people reading this book will flip to the chapters on
snoring and sleep apnea, there are a host of other problems that
can keep you from getting good sleep—some serious and some
not so serious. Just as specific risk factors indicate a greater chance
of problems such as a heart attack, osteoporosis, or diabetes, the
following risk factors indicate who is likely to have a sleep-related disorder:

TABLE 1.5	

Common Sleep Disturbances

Do any of these common problems affect your sleep? If so, talk with
your doctor about solutions.

no	Many arousals during a night's sleep
no	Awakening in the middle of the night
no	Difficulty in getting to sleep
no	Reduction in total sleep time
no	Long awakenings (ten minutes or longer) during sleep
no	Restless legs or arms (jerks or movement) during sleep
yes	Awakening feeling exhausted and foggy
no	Frightening nightmares
?	Gasping, choking, or pauses in breathing during sleep
no	A feeling of creeping sensations in legs while lying down
no	A feeling of chest tightness or congestion
no	Difficulty in breathing
yes	Nasal congestion at night
no	Tossing, turning, and an inability to relax
yes	Mouth breathing
no	Frequent awakenings from loud snoring
no	Frequent awakenings and a feeling of gasping for breath

....

- Age

- Obesity

- Abnormalities in the upper airway, nose, or throat (such as enlarged tonsils)

- Cigarette smoking

- Chronic respiratory or cardiac ailment

Go through the checklist in Table 1.5, and see what might be causing your particular sleep problem. If your sleep problem stems from too much caffeine or an inability to relax, set aside the worries of the day before bedtime and avoid caffeine after noon each day. Yet if your problem seems more serious, ask your doctor for a referral to a sleep clinic for a medical evaluation. (Table 1.6 has a list of some common sleep-related disorders.)

TABLE 1.6	

Sleep-Related Disorders

Insomnia—disruption of the sleep cycle with difficulty getting to sleep, or difficulty staying asleep

Snoring—audible sound that happens during sleep when the soft parts of the throat vibrate

Sleep apnea—potentially life-threatening problem in which a person stops breathing as a result of relaxed or excessive tissue blocking the airway

Narcolepsy—a genetic disorder that causes a persistent and insatiable need to sleep

Restless legs syndrome—a creeping, crawling sensation in the legs (and sometimes in the arms) that creates an irresistible urge to move

SNOOZE YOU CAN USE

What happens if you feel tired and try to relax yet still cannot achieve restful sleep? Talk with your doctor. If your doctor suspects that you might have a sleep disorder, you might be referred for a sleep study called a *polysomnography* (see Chapter 5), especially if you have excessive daytime sleepiness or a problem staying asleep. The sleep study will help determine if you have pure snoring, obstructive sleep apnea, restless legs syndrome, or another problem. All these disorders require specific therapy that your doctor will prescribe.

CHAPTER 2

Snoring: The Noisy Thief

Idon't snore and if I do, it surely isn't very loud or often."
Ben was so convinced that his wife was overreacting
when she made an appointment to have his snoring evaluated at the Cleveland Clinic that he started to walk out the clinic door.

If you're like Ben and don't think you snore, ask your bed
partner, housemates, or family members, for they usually know for
sure. If you do snore, it's time to take it seriously. Snoring not only
is disruptive to your sleep, your daytime performance, and your
family relations, but it also often sets you up as an object of ridicule
and makes you an unwanted guest on weekend camping trips. In
addition to its social implications, snoring can often be an early
warning sign of more serious problems such as obstructive sleep
apnea (OSA)—when breathing actually stops during sleep.

Look at the following common snoring-related complaints
patients have shared:

- It drives my wife from the bedroom.

- My girlfriend won't marry me.

- Even my dog leaves my bedroom at night when I snore.

- My kids won't have their friends spend the night because my snoring embarrasses them.

- I snore so loudly at movies and at church, they've asked me to leave.

- I had such poor sleep from snoring that I fell asleep during a business meeting with my boss.

- My friends said I could not come on the fishing trip because of my snoring.

- Snoring seems to disrupt my sleep so much that I can hardly keep my eyes open to drive home from work.

- I had a serious car wreck because I fell asleep while driving.

ASK YOUR FAMILY

"Ben's snoring is so loud it even keeps our dog up all night," Janis said. "Especially if Ben has allergies from springtime pollen or has a few beers while watching TV, my daughter and I know it's going to be a long night with no sleep."

Bed partners or family members can often provide important information regarding the loudness and frequency of snoring and factors that worsen snoring such as position (lying on the back or side), cigarette smoking, or allergies that cause nasal congestion. They are also usually the ones who demand answers, encouraging the snorer to seek help. After all, if you are asleep, you may not be aware of the noise you make each night.

Through the years, bed partners have taken it upon themselves to solve the snoring problem, using such obscure remedies as stuffing a cloth in the snorer's mouth. Snorers have claimed fractured ribs from getting hard pokes during the night by a bed partner in an attempt to jolt the snorer and quiet the noise. In an extreme case of listener annoyance, the gunslinger John Wesley Hardin is remarked to have fatally shot a loud snorer in the next room.

Before you stuff a washcloth in your bed partner's mouth or load your gun (or worry that someone may try to do this to "end" your snoring problem!), keep reading. We want you to understand all about snoring—why it occurs, who is at risk, and even possible deleterious health consequences that can develop within this large set of people we call "snorers."

NOT FOR MEN ONLY

If you are a woman reading this, you may be thinking, "Snoring is such a 'man thing.'" Up to a certain age, this is true, as *more than 60 percent of all men ages thirty-five to sixty-five* snore. Men are more prone to snoring for a variety of reasons, from hormonal effects on the upper-airway muscles, differences in the distribution of body fat between men and women, and variations in the anatomy and function of the upper airways (the nose and throat at the back of the tongue). However, the statistics change at around age sixty, with the number of women snorers increasing dramatically because of hormonal changes at menopause and body fat distribution. The incidence of snoring sometimes diminishes in men after age sixty-five, yet it remains stable in women.

While the snorer may sleep seemingly undisturbed by the noises she emits, the sound levels of snoring, recorded to be as high as 88 decibels, can be as loud as the diesel engine one hears when sitting in the back of an old bus. These nocturnal sounds not only are an annoying nuisance to the sleepless bed partner, but also can interrupt one's sexual relationship. For bed partners, how sexy is it to lie in bed and listen to your mate continually make thunderous roars, gasps, and sighs throughout the night, and then to have both of you suffer with the consequences of sleep loss, fatigue, and an inability to concentrate on love making?

More than 42 percent of men with OSA are impotent. Studies have consistently revealed that men who snore heavily and have OSA may lose their sexual urges because of fatigue or depression, or both, just as some depressed people lose their appetite for food.

Problems maintaining a penile erection can be the result of fatigue or coincidental vascular or neurologic abnormalities in men who have OSA. These men may also have other medical problems such as high blood pressure, diabetes mellitus, or increased age. Some men taking medications for hypertension or depression may experience impotence. Treatment of the OSA, a possible underlying cause of the high blood pressure or depression, may get rid of or reduce the need for these drugs and improve sexual function.

Snoring is an extremely serious social and public health hazard and may cause poor quality of sleep, changes in the sleep-wake cycle, and lower levels of oxygen in the blood as a result of OSA. Because of restless sleep and frequent awakenings, there is diminished daytime alertness, resulting in dramatic alterations in mood, effectiveness, and energy. You know what one poor night's sleep can do to your personality and performance. But consider a snorer and his bed partner who have not slept soundly in years.

WHY ALL THE FUSS?

While you may feel isolated from family and friends because of your snoring, you can relax because you have great company. The following statistics are enough to disturb anyone's sleep:

- Some 45 percent of all normal adults snore occasionally.

- Forty million Americans snore habitually; 20 to 30 million more experience sleep-related problems.

- Snoring exists at all age levels and may occur with greater intensity as we age.

- Twenty percent of men between ages thirty and thirty-five and 5 percent of young women snore.

- Because of changes in hormones and fat distribution at menopause, by age sixty, 40 percent of women snore habitually.

- By age sixty, 60 percent of men snore habitually.

- Snoring may be caused by obesity, heavy alcohol drinking, cigarette smoking, hormones, facial size, genetics, and age.

- Snoring is associated with morning headaches, restless legs during sleep, mood swings, choking sensations, impotence, hypertension, heart disease, stroke, and even death.

- Ten to 50 percent of those who snore have OSA, which can cause early death (see Chapter 3).

As the data from comprehensive studies show, snoring is more common in men than in women, and it is increasingly more common with increased age and weight. While airway diseases such as asthma get great attention, the number of adults who snore is greater than the number of those who have asthma. Interestingly, of middle-aged and older men, those who snore are probably as common as those who smoke cigarettes.

Recently, scientists have attempted to determine whether snoring is associated with an increased risk of heart attacks or strokes and of sudden death. The jury is now in, and in spite of some limitations in the studies, the good news is that snoring is *not* an independent risk factor for heart attacks or strokes. Sophisticated research and subsequent reviews of sleep studies suggest that when there is an association between snoring and cardiovascular disease, undiagnosed OSA—not pure snoring—may have accounted for the increased risk.

THE CAUSES OF SNORING

Now that you know snoring affects millions of people and may be associated with serious problems if left untreated, it will help to understand what causes this problem. If you've ever gone whitewater rafting, you know that the river rumbles and roars as it twists and turns down a mountainside. The sound of the water changes depending on such factors as speed, wind, and obstacles such as rocks that impede the flow. Similarly, strong winds blowing between skyscrapers in narrow alleyways will produce whistling or howling sounds. You might compare these noises with the sounds we call snoring.

Over the past couple of years, fascinating research has shown exactly how snoring occurs. The muscles supporting the opening of the upper airway in the back of the throat relax during sleep. Extra tissue in the palate and uvula—the fleshy piece between the tonsils—vibrates with each breath, and these vibrations actually cause the sound of snoring. In some people, the airway has a tendency to close at any point. Narrowing of the airway will cause turbulence and the noises of snoring (see Figure 2.1).

During sleep, snorers experience a limitation of airflow along with turbulence at the entrance to the respiratory system (see page 9). This narrowing and vibrating is caused by structural factors such as fat deposits around the upper airway or neurological problems such as a lack of coordination between the muscles that keep open the upper airway and the main breathing muscles such as the diaphragm. This happens when the upper-airway muscles relax yet the diaphragm continues to work. Snoring can occur when you breathe in or breathe out and whether you breathe through your nose or your mouth.

Interestingly, snorers may be predestined to snore from birth. Using such imaging techniques as a computerized tomography (CT) and magnetic resonance imaging (MRI), researchers have found that snorers have specific abnormalities in the anatomy of the upper airway that are different from nonsnorers. These differences may be in the bony structures of the face and at various sites along the air passage from the back of the nose to the base of the tongue just above the vocal cords. These images show that typically the size of the upper airway is smaller in people who snore than it is in people who do not snore. Abnormalities causing a narrowing of the upper airway could be from a broken or crooked nose, which decreases the airway size; obstructions in the nasal airways from swollen mucous membranes; or extra fat deposits around the upper airway that cut down on airway size.

It is the upper-airway dimensions and the decreased activity of

FIGURE 2.1

AN ANATOMICAL VIEW SHOWING WHERE NO RIGID
SUPPORT EXISTS AND WHERE SNORING ORIGINATES

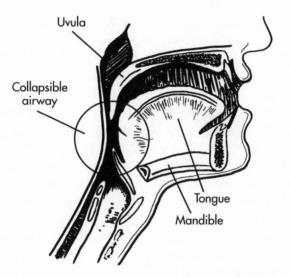

the supporting muscles during sleep that predispose to airway closure during sleep and the subsequent snoring or sleep apnea.

THANK YOUR UPPER AIRWAY

Usually the only time you think about your upper airway is when
you have a cold. You can't breathe and have difficulty swallowing,
and the constant drainage of mucus makes you choke. However, this
part of your respiratory system is a very complicated and important
structure that does some amazing things for which you should be
grateful. Your upper airway is responsible for voice production,
swallowing, keeping the back of the throat clear of food and mucus,
and preparing the air you breathe to go into your lungs.

Within the upper airway are about twenty muscles that are
responsible for carrying out these daily functions, as well as for

maintaining the opening of the airway, even when factors tend to make it close or collapse. Some muscles in the walls of the upper airway and in the surrounding tissues must keep the airway open as you breathe in and out.

When you are awake, your airways do not collapse or narrow because of activity of the airway dilator muscles. If you snore, this activity increases during wakefulness to overcome the narrowing. Yet problems arise when you hit the bed and fall asleep. During NREM sleep (see page 7), the activity of the airway dilator muscles is decreased, and during REM sleep (page 7), the activity is almost completely gone. This is why sleep researchers have found that snoring usually worsens during REM sleep.

Although the exact point of airway collapse is different among people, finding out the exact place where your airway is narrowing will help your doctor prescribe the precise treatment or "cure" for your snoring.

COMMON RISK FACTORS

As you will learn in Chapters 5 to 8, the treatment for snoring is easy and effective once the exact cause of the problem is identified. If you snore, you may notice that a recent weight gain, even as small as 10 percent of your baseline body weight, has worsened the problem. This may be caused by the deposition of fat in the neck around the upper airway, which adds to the narrowing of the airway and increases the tendency to snore. Collar size and the increased risk of OSA are discussed in Chapter 3.

Mac, a thirty-nine-year-old attorney, had never snored until he fractured his ankle in a company softball game and was on crutches for eight weeks. While Mac used to run each evening to keep his weight normal, now he was forced to sit in a chair after work and watch TV. This inactivity combined with extra TV snacks caused Mac to gain fifteen pounds in just two months, and that's when the snoring began. When his wife awoke him four times in one hour for disturbing her sleep, they knew it was time to seek medical help.

After performing a physical examination and some tests described in Chapter 5, Mac's doctor believed that his snoring could be managed easily with one easy cure: weight loss. Mac's sudden weight gain had increased his waistline and his neck size, as excess fatty tissue had collected around his upper airway, leading to snoring. Losing the fifteen pounds by using the suggestions in Chapter 6 helped Mac get back to his normal weight—and to normal sleep without snoring. Now Mac knows that staying at a normal weight will keep his snoring at bay and allow him and his wife to get restful sleep.

While obesity is a key risk factor for snoring, there are also other environmental and genetic risk factors that influence snoring, including cigarette smoking, respiratory disease, allergies, or obstructions such as polyps or swollen tonsils. Knowing the common risk factors for snoring can aid you in determining the root cause of your snoring problem, as well as its severity.

Heavy alcohol use is a key risk factor for snoring and certain medications such as muscle relaxants, tranquilizers, and sleeping pills can also worsen snoring (and perhaps lead to sleep apnea) by inducing relaxation of the pharyngeal muscles. Smoking is another practice that increases the chance of snoring, possibly as a result of the irritative effects of the smoke on the airway, with pharyngeal narrowing caused by swelling of the tissues exposed to the smoke. Nasal congestion caused by either seasonal or perennial allergies may also aggravate snoring. Allergic or infectious rhinitis, sinusitis, a cold, or injury can cause nasal obstruction and the subsequent snoring. If you are a mouth breather because of nasal congestion, the chances that you snore are even greater. (Treatment for nasal congestion is discussed in Chapter 7.)

As you read the specific risk factors in Table 2.1, you will realize that some, including age, gender, and chronic respiratory disease, cannot be changed. The good news is that other risk factors, including obesity, allergies and nasal congestion, sleep positions, exercise, diet, heavy alcohol use, smoking cigarettes, and using certain medications, can and must be changed.

TABLE 2.1	

Risk Factors for Snoring

Sex (male)

Age

Obesity

Short, fat neck

Poor tone (lack of tightness) in the muscles of the tongue and throat

Allergies, respiratory problems, or mouth breathing

Upper-airway obstruction (enlarged tonsils or adenoids, polyps, deviated septum)

Sleep positions (sleeping on back)

Heavy meals before bedtime

Certain medications such as antihistamines, sleeping pills, and tranquilizers

Certain illnesses such as hypothyroidism

Cigarette smoking

Alcohol use close to bedtime

Menopause (women)

FINDING ANSWERS

If you snore, your bed partner may have already suggested (or demanded!) that you seek medical help. In our clinics, we have experienced that sometimes the snorer is literally dragged to the doctor's office with demands of "fix this problem . . . now!" The bed partner can usually provide excellent information on the type of snoring, including the frequency. When the snorer is not accompanied to the doctor's examination by his or her bed partner, it is important for the physician to get more information from that person by asking the following questions:

• How severe is the snoring?

- Does it cause disruption with family and friends?

- How long has the snoring been a problem?

- Does it occur every night or occasionally, such as when the snorer has a cold or when his allergies are acting up?

- Is snoring mainly a problem after drinking alcohol in the evening?

- Does snoring occur only when the person lies on her back?

- Is the snoring associated with increased moving around in bed during sleep?

- Are there quiet, breath-holding spells accompanied by sounds of gagging, choking, gasping, or snoring, and then resumed snoring?

EVALUATING YOUR SNORING PROBLEM

The ear-nose-throat (ENT) specialist (otolaryngologist) may be the first specialist who does an evaluation to discover your snoring problem and to prescribe the subsequent cure. Sometimes the first doctor may be the family practitioner, the pediatrician, a general internist, or a pulmonologist. During this evaluation, the doctor will take a thorough history, highlighting the questions listed on pages 24–25, as there are specific therapeutic remedies, depending on the responses.

Your doctor will also perform the following:

- A complete physical examination, focusing on the nose, throat, neck, and abdomen

- A measurement of your neck, particularly if it is short and fat

- A thorough check to see if you have nasal polyps, swollen turbinates, or a deviated septum

- A check for signs of old fractures of the nose, as well as enlargement of the tongue or elongation of the palate with swelling of the uvula

- An assessment of your jawbone from the side view to consider its size, angulation, and whether or not there is an overbite

To perform some of the tests necessary to identify the root of your snoring, the ENT surgeon may use a special telescope, a *fiberoptic laryngoscope*, to look in more detail at the nasopharynx, oropharynx, and hypopharynx—or the entrance to the respiratory system (see Table 2.2).

The extent and nature of the crowding in your upper airway will tend to validate the complaints of the listener (usually a bed partner) whose suffering prompted the visit to the physician. A large tongue pushing back on the oropharynx and a swollen, reddened, bulky uvula are common findings in people with loud snoring.

The doctor may also decide to order blood tests to evaluate the function of your thyroid gland. A low-functioning thyroid secretes less active hormone into the blood, which predisposes you to obesity and may change the pattern of breathing.

Special radiological images such as CT scans of the sinuses or of the soft tissues of the neck may be ordered. These will allow the doctor to see in more detail the nature of the nasal congestion or the narrowing in the throat. Use of these additional tests will depend on your overall medical history, the physical examination, and what the doctor believes is necessary to better evaluate your problem. Keep in mind that the doctor should have a clear-cut therapeutic or diagnostic reason for all tests performed.

TABLE 2.2

The Entrance to the Respiratory System

Nasopharynx—the region behind the turbinates and the hard palate
Oropharynx—subdivided into the region behind the palate and the region behind the tongue
Hypopharynx—the region from the base of the tongue to the larynx

THE ROLE OF THE SLEEP STUDY

One of the biggest decisions to be made when you are evaluated for snoring is whether or not a sleep study should be done. *Polysomnography*, merely a technical term for sleep study, is performed in a special laboratory. As you will learn in Chapter 5, the sleep study can be a lifesaving evaluation and can sometimes be done in the privacy of your own home.

If you snore and wonder whether a sleep study might benefit you, the following questions deserve emphasis:

- Do you have any of the symptoms listed in Table 3.1 on page 30?

- Do you have headaches upon awakening?

- Do you have abnormal heart rhythms?

- Has the doctor tested your oxygen levels and found them to be low?

- Are you sleepy during the day after what you thought was a good night's sleep?

- Do you have problems functioning during the daytime, such as having difficulty with memory or concentration?

- Does your bed partner describe hearing you snore, yet hearing intermittent pauses in your snoring possibly caused by a cessation of breathing?

- Do you awaken during the night for no clear reason?

- Do you awaken frequently during the night to urinate?

EARLY DIAGNOSIS LEADS TO EFFECTIVE TREATMENT

If you replied yes to any of these questions and if you snore, polysomnography will help determine whether or not you have "pure" snoring or OSA. This distinction is important because the treatment is different for each problem. Polysomnography will assess the actual quality of your sleep using a combination of special tests, explained in Chapter 5. These tests provide important data that define the time it takes you to fall asleep, the duration of your sleep, and the time you spend in the different stages of sleep. Brief arousals, full awakenings, and movements are also recorded to determine the severity of the fragmentation of sleep, which might account for daytime sleepiness and other symptoms. Most important, the pattern of breathing including airflow at the nose and mouth along with the movements of your chest wall and abdomen is recorded to determine the occurrence of apneas.

After this thorough assessment, the sleep specialist and your doctor will work together to make recommendations for a snoring cure. If your doctor does not believe that a sleep study is warranted, you will be given specific nonsurgical or surgical options for stopping snoring, as defined in Chapters 7 and 8.

THE SNORING CURE WILL WORK

No matter how severe your snoring problem is, there is hope. You do not have to suffer night after night, waking up because a bed partner pokes you in the ribs for snoring or feeling exhausted because upper-airway obstructions or apneas cause fragmented sleep. Especially with the newer methods of evaluating snoring and its root causes, along with the surgical and nonsurgical "cures," every man and woman can know with confidence that even as they age, they can enjoy good-quality sleep with reduced daytime sleepiness. Starting the easy steps for treatment and prevention of further snoring problems will allow you to sleep like a baby again and enjoy your life more fully.

CHAPTER 3

Sleep Apnea: More Than a Nuisance

A s you learned in Chapter 2, snoring is caused by vibration of the soft parts of the throat while you are breathing in and out during sleep. Sometimes, this noise is continuous with almost every breath. Or, in some people, the noise may be sporadic with periods of breath holding. These periods when breathing stops are called *apneas* and are caused by obstruction of the upper airway at the level of the uvula or base of the tongue. Apneas may be interrupted by a brief arousal that does not result in complete awakening; in fact, you may not even realize you were disturbed during sleep. Yet arousals represent a characteristic change in the brain waves that lasts only a few seconds and is noticeable on *electroencephalographic* recordings (see page 54).

While daytime sleepiness has been estimated to occur in 5 percent of the population, as many as 30 to 40 percent of those with sleep apnea have daytime fatigue. As a forty-one-year-old woman who was recently diagnosed with obstructive sleep apnea (OSA) said, "I go to bed tired, I awaken tired, and I'm tired all day. I'm beginning to think that being tired all the time is just normal for me." Being tired during daytime hours is *not* normal and can be resolved if you get to the root of the sleep-related problem.

Those with OSA may also have other very serious symptoms after what they thought was a good night's sleep, as the arousals disturb or even ruin the normally refreshing nature of sleep. Low oxygen levels, which result when blockages prevent air from getting to the lungs, also affect the brain and heart.

As with snoring, the statistics on OSA are disturbing. Consider the following:

- In adults, as many as 10 to 50 percent of those who snore have sleep apnea. (Millions of those who snore have not been diagnosed with this serious problem yet have serious symptoms, as listed in Table 3.1.)

- In adults, OSA is more common than asthma.

TABLE 3.1	

Common Symptoms of Obstructive Sleep Apnea (OSA)*

Morning headaches
High blood pressure
Dry mouth
Sore throat upon awakening
Depression
Concentration problems
Memory failure
Impotence
Excessive daytime sleepiness
Restless sleep (increased movements)
Choking sensations
Frequent awakenings
Irregular heart rhythm
Bed-wetting

*Some children with bed-wetting (enuresis) have OSA. Some people who grind their teeth during sleep, a problem known as bruxism, have OSA.

- People with more than twenty apneas (complete obstructions) per hour of sleep may have a greater risk of dying from cardiac rhythm and rate disturbances and complications of high blood pressure such as stroke and heart attacks than people with fewer apneas.

- Up to two-thirds of the people who have OSA are overweight.

- Analysis of data from several studies suggests that the association between snoring and high blood pressure, coronary disease, and strokes may be related to obesity and the presence of OSA.

And the statistics only become more exhausting. Some people with OSA awaken frequently to urinate and think their arousals are from urological problems. Actually the real cause of their sleep disruption is OSA. OSA is also found in one-third of people with hypertension, as well as in those who have nasal blockages or obstructions, enlargements of the tonsils or adenoids, or a misplaced jawbone. Allergies and mouth breathing play a large role as risk factors for OSA, as well.

UPPER-AIRWAY PROBLEMS

"It never fails that just when I finally relax, ready to drift off to dreamland and recharge my battery, I start to cough and sneeze. Or, my nose begins to feel stuffy and congested, and my chest feels tight, and I begin to wheeze." Candy's sleep problem of unending snoring seemed to start with her constant and poorly managed allergic rhinitis.

A broad spectrum of breathing problems can occur during sleep. These problems range from noisy snoring stemming from the vibration of the structures in the pharynx caused by the turbulence of airflow, to apnea or the cessation of breathing brought about by complete closure of the upper airway. In between are other problems that most sleep experts view as a sort of continuum.

Perhaps the word *apnea* is foreign to you, but in simplest terms it literally means *without breathing*. Apnea is used to describe an interruption of airflow that lasts at least ten seconds. While there are three different kinds of apneas, the most common type is *obstructive*, accounting for 65 percent of all apneas. During this type of apnea there is no airflow from the nose and mouth to the lungs because the entrance to the trachea is completely blocked by different structures in the pharynx that have collapsed. While the structures are closed, the respiratory muscles continue to make efforts to get air into the lungs.

A much less common type of apnea is called *central*. Central apnea accounts for about 10 percent of all the apneas. In this situation, there is no airflow because the respiratory muscles receive no stimulation from the central nervous system. A *mixed apnea* is one that begins as a *central* event but then becomes *obstructive* during attempts to breathe. The lack of stimulation of respiratory muscles results in no airflow, without which the airway collapses and air is unable to pass through once effort begins.

Other partial occlusions of the pharyngeal airway, called *hypopneas*, can also occur. With a hypopnea, airflow is decreased by 50 percent, accompanied by a 4 percent fall in blood oxygen level. Hypopneas, like the apnea, may end with an arousal. These arousals may not be long enough or severe enough to cause complete awakening but are sufficient to ruin sleep if frequent. In some cases, the changes in airflow in the upper airway are extremely subtle.

The *upper-airway resistance syndrome* (UARS) is still another sleep-disordered breathing problem in which there are repeated, very brief arousals associated with increased airway resistance due to some narrowing of the airway. A person with UARS may have periods of crescendo snoring, which is characterized by a noise that gradually gets louder. At the end of each episode of crescendo snoring, arousal occurs, along with an abrupt decrease in upper-airway resistance. Snoring may subside briefly until another episode occurs. The good news is that with UARS, there are *no* significant drops in oxygen level. Yet, as with hypopnea or apnea, the arousals from UARS cause fragmented sleep and daytime sleepiness as a result of the sleep deprivation. Many hypopneas and UARS events cause the same symptoms as full-blown OSA.

Snoring, discussed in detail in the previous chapter, is often the first warning signal of sleep-disordered breathing. Other clues, as mentioned earlier, indicate that something more serious than snoring is taking place.

A TYPICAL PORTRAIT OF SLEEP APNEA

For years, Rick, a fifty-three-year-old computer program analyst, had interrupted sleep caused by constant "elbowing" by his wife, who was trying to stop his thunderous snoring. His nighttime snoring worsened to the point that his wife began to sleep in the guest bedroom to get a good night's rest. However, what particularly frightened her were the episodes of apparent breath holding Rick was experiencing during sleep. These apneas lasted up to eighty seconds each, and she told of lying awake many nights just waiting for these to happen so she could jolt Rick into breathing again.

Not only was her own lack of sleep frustrating, but also Rick's wife was tired of his inability to stay awake at family functions, during symphony concerts, or at their daughter's ballet recital. Rick was personally concerned about a new symptom: severe headaches that started to occur regularly every morning. At work, he began to consume huge amounts of coffee or caffeinated cola drinks to keep himself awake at the computer monitor.

When his son read about sleep apnea on the Internet, he encouraged his parents to go to a sleep disorders center for help. After a series of consultations and sleep testing, Rick found out that he did have sleep apnea. (The symptoms of sleep apnea are discussed in detail on page 30, and include loud, annoying snoring that is punctuated by quiet spells or cessation of breathing called apneas, which are ended by an audible resumption of breathing and continuation of snoring.)

After talking with some close business colleagues, Rick soon discovered that another computer analyst in his firm had the same problem and was successfully treated with nasal continuous positive airway pressure (CPAP) (see page 94). This involves wearing a custom-fit mask with a tight-fitting seal over the nose during sleep. The mask is attached by a flexible hose to a pump. Essentially, this device blows air into the nose to keep the airway from collapsing during sleep. Nasal CPAP does not cure OSA but controls the symptoms by preventing narrowing of the airway and the associated arousals. Not wearing the device for even one night can cause a recurrence of the daytime sleepiness and other symptoms such as headaches that occur in the morning.

Rick used nasal CPAP for a short time and was amazed at how much better he felt. His headaches soon disappeared, and his alertness and energy level increased. His wife even moved back into their bedroom because he no longer snored. Also, his fishing buddies agreed that Rick could rejoin the group and come with them on overnight cruises—but only if he brought along his portable battery system to run the nasal CPAP machine on the boat.

Rick is now a committed "sleep activist" and speaks regularly

---

TABLE 3.2

Common Risk Factors for Obstructive Sleep Apnea

Gender: males twice as common as females

Obesity: more than 120% of ideal body weight

Neck size: collar larger than 17 inches in men and 15 inches in women

Enlarged tonsils

Nasal septum deviation

Small jawbone or backward displacement of jawbone

Glandular disorders: hypothyroidism, acromegaly

Genetic predisposition: family history

Specific genetic disease: Down's syndrome (an uncommon genetic disease, with the apnea possibly associated with abnormal facial or upper-airway anatomy)

Medicines or drugs: see Table 3.3

---

to support groups in South Florida for people with sleep apnea, telling them of new treatments that can change their lives.

IDENTIFYING THE PERSON WITH OBSTRUCTIVE SLEEP APNEA

Just as there are specific risk factors that contribute to the snoring problem, there are also *common* risk factors that can help to identify the person with OSA, as shown in Table 3.2. Other factors associated with OSA are listed in Tables 3.3 and 3.4.

TABLE 3.3

Medicines or Drugs That Can Worsen Snoring or Cause Obstructive Sleep Apnea

Alcohol
Hypnotics (sleeping pills)
Narcotic pain relievers
Tranquilizers

TABLE 3.4

Genetic Diseases Associated with Obstructive Sleep Apnea

Down's syndrome
Apert's syndrome, Treacher Collins syndrome, achondroplasia (extremely rare genetic diseases)

SLEEP APNEA: A SERIOUS SLEEP DISORDER

The National Commission of Sleep Disorders Research was established by Congress in 1988. This commission reports that each year the lives of millions of Americans are disrupted, disturbed, or destroyed by the consequences of sleep disorders. Of all the sleep disorders discussed, including narcolepsy, nocturnal myoclonus, and insomnia, the most serious sleep disorder is sleep apnea because of airflow obstruction and cessation of respiration.

Even though affected persons and family members might consider sleep apnea bothersome, it is a common and potentially fatal disorder, with adverse effects on multiple organ systems in the body, especially the heart. These adverse effects can cause mild to severe organ dysfunction. Fortunately, various forms of treatment are currently available, as you will learn in Chapters 6 through 8. Of the treatments available, however, nasal CPAP is the most common and effective one used today. The CPAP machine, by way of a mask worn during sleep, maintains a positive pressure inside the airway during respiration. It acts as a support to prevent further narrowing or collapse of the airway and actually increases the size of the airway behind the palate and at the back of the tongue. Nasal CPAP not only relieves the symptom of excessive daytime sleepiness but also is effective in improving and reducing the severity of medical problems associated with sleep apnea.

Direct Effects and Medical Complications

The medical complications of untreated OSA occur because of the *direct effects* of the periodic blockages in the upper airway. These direct effects include low blood oxygen levels, the production of large changes in the pressure inside the chest cavity, and arousals from sleep that occur almost every time the airway narrows.

The problems or medical complications associated with untreated sleep apnea are as follows:

• **Systemic hypertension**—high blood pressure, which causes an increased risk of heart disease, strokes, kidney failure, and poor circulation

- **Left-sided heart failure**—inability of the heart to pump the blood adequately, causing shortness of breath, fatigue, and poor ability to exercise

- **Pulmonary hypertension**—elevated blood pressure in the lungs, associated with shortness of breath, chest pain, and increased mortality

- **Arrhythmias**—irregularity of the heart rate

- **Ischemic heart disease**—angina pectoris (chest pain) and heart attacks (myocardial infarction) caused by an insufficient supply of blood to the heart

- **Stroke**—damage to the brain caused by blockage of blood flow or bleeding

- **Increased mortality**

- **Excessive daytime sleepiness**

- **Impaired daytime performance**

- **Personality changes**

Increased Mortality Rate

Earlier studies have shown that OSA patients have an increased mortality rate, as much as ten times higher than normal. The cause for the high mortality rate is thought to be a combination of cardiovascular and cerebrovascular events. Along with OSA, there are other factors present, such as advanced age, obesity, cardiovascular diseases, and stroke. While landmark studies found that using nasal CPAP reduces or normalizes the blood pressure in the hypertensive patient with OSA, it does not lower the blood pressure in the person who does not have hypertension associated with OSA. Unfortunately, researchers are not sure whether the reduction in blood pressure is primarily a result of the effect of nasal CPAP, or whether the people who use nasal CPAP have also changed their lifestyle, such as losing weight, increasing exercise, and changing dietary habits.

Few studies on OSA have focused on mortality. One sophisticated study reviewed 246 untreated patients with OSA over an eight-year period. Those with a moderate or severe degree of OSA had a mortality rate of 37 percent, while those with milder disease had a mortality rate of only 4 percent. Other closely related studies demonstrated a higher mortality rate in those treated conservatively with weight loss, compared to those treated with tracheostomy.

While sudden death can occur in OSA patients, the contribution of hypertension and cardiovascular (heart attack) and cerebrovascular (stroke) disease to mortality in OSA has not been well established.

Problems in Brain Function

Persons with OSA may feel a bit foggy and dense during daytime hours. Impairment in intellectual performance (attentiveness, alertness, memory) is found in more than half of those with OSA. The major problems experienced are deficits in thinking, perception, memory, communication, and the ability to learn new information. These deficits can result in high anxiety, confusion, irritability, and often depression. The symptoms are then magnified by their effects on interpersonal relationships and work performance.

Cognitive impairment can be seen in OSA patients who do not develop low oxygen levels in the blood, or *hypoxemia*, at night. In these patients, the problems with function are attributable to the poor sleep or frequent awakening resulting from the arousals that end the episodes of upper-airway narrowing.

Automobile Deaths

Automobile accidents are the third leading cause of death in the United States, with 2 million accidents occurring yearly, resulting in 45,000 deaths. Sleep apnea has been linked to automobile accidents. A study examining auto accidents and the number of accidents in which the driver was at fault found that those with sleep apnea had a six to seven times greater chance of being in an accident and being the cause of the crash. Some of the accidents occurred after the people fell asleep or "blacked out" at the wheel.

Numerous reports have shown that OSA poses an elevated risk of falling asleep while driving, being involved in non-alcohol-related accidents, and crossing the center line, resulting in a crash. Poor ability to maintain concentration and slow reaction times are central to this problem, resulting in impairment and poor judgment in operating a vehicle. Individuals with sleep apnea have a higher percentage of more severe, often high-speed crashes, head-on collisions, or hitting a stationary object at high speed.

More than 90 percent of those with OSA report having excessive daytime sleepiness. Comprehensive studies also have shown that 60 to 85 percent of those with a chief complaint of excessive daytime sleepiness have OSA as the cause.

Whether people with sleep apnea should be allowed to drive or not presents a legal issue. The laws governing the doctor's obligation in this situation are ambiguous and vary from state to state. Ethically, doctors are obliged to suggest that if you are drowsy during daytime hours, you should not operate dangerous machinery, boats, trucks, or cars.

SLEEP APNEA MAY WORSEN OTHER AILMENTS

If you have been going to the doctor with a variety of unresolved cardiac problems, ask about testing for sleep apnea. Especially if the doctor has suggested that you may have coronary artery disease, congestive heart failure, hypertension, cardiac arrhythmias, strokes, or cerebral infarction, sleep apnea may be a big contributor. Sleep apnea can also be problematic in otherwise well people, or it may further worsen the health status in someone with underlying disease.

In the event that your snoring problem is actually OSA, you

need to seek medical attention soon. The next steps in diagnosis and treatment are discussed in Chapters 5 to 8. But by far the most important step is the one that you must take yourself—talk to the doctor about your snoring problem, get a thorough evaluation at a sleep center, if necessary, and start treatment immediately.

CHAPTER 4

The Snoring Cure: An Overview

A fter reading the first three chapters, perhaps you are beginning to understand how snoring is much more than noise. Perhaps you also see why taking charge of a snoring problem is essential—for better sleep, increased energy, and outstanding daytime performance, as well as to avoid the deleterious health consequences of obstructive sleep apnea (OSA) such as high blood pressure, heart disease, and stroke.

The four steps to cure snoring will help you finally put an end to this disruptive and unhealthy noise:

Step 1: Get an accurate diagnosis. Find out the cause of your snoring and resulting fatigue, such as OSA or another serious health problem (see Chapter 5).

Step 2: Maintain a normal weight. Many times, losing weight can greatly reduce or even end snoring and possibly OSA. While continuous positive airway pressure (see page 94) is the treatment of choice for OSA, it is not a cure. Permanent weight loss may result in a cure, so check out which recommendations are best for permanent weight loss (see Chapter 6).

Step 3:   Try nonsurgical treatments. There are a myriad of treatment measures to try that may stop your snoring tonight. Some
can be purchased over the counter; some may need to be pre-
scribed by your doctor; others may involve changing the way you
sleep. Chapter 7 describes known and little-known treatments that
can work.

Step 4:   Use the surgical snoring cures. For some serious cases of
snoring, you may be able to opt for surgery. Chapter 8 explains the
latest surgical snoring cures, including who is a candidate, the costs
and preparation, how the procedure is done, and the health risks
involved.

The overall goal with the **four-step cure** is to become aware
of snoring as a serious health concern and then to use the four successful ways to stop this problem altogether. The program repre-
sents the most credible and practical snoring solutions on the mar-
ket and can easily be implemented, starting today!

CHAPTER 5

Step 1: Get an Accurate Diagnosis

While more than 55 percent of those who snore never even discuss this with their physician, talking about this common problem and getting an accurate diagnosis are the first steps to curing snoring. The doctor is crucial for determining the exact cause of the problem, as well as testing to see if the problem is "pure" snoring or obstructive sleep apnea.

GETTING THE PRECISE DIAGNOSIS

The doctor you select for the initial evaluation may be one of the health care professionals listed in Table 5.1. After a thorough physical examination, the physician may refer you to a sleep disorder specialist. This doctor is familiar with the signs and symptoms of obstructive sleep apnea, as well as a host of other sleep disorders. The sleep disorder specialist will find making the diagnosis relatively simple and will promptly decide if you need to have a confirmatory sleep study (polysomnography).

TABLE 5.1	

Health Care Professionals

Primary care physician: This doctor is a general practitioner, a family practice doctor, pediatrician, or internist who has completed three years of training after medical school graduation.

Allergist: An allergist is a pediatrician or internist who has taken additional training to qualify as a specialist in allergy and immunology after completing training in a primary specialty.

Internist: A doctor who specializes in internal medicine, the study of diseases in adults, particularly those related to internal organs, and who has completed three years of training after medical school.

Otolaryngologist: An ear-nose-throat specialist who treats problems with the ears, nose, throat, and related structures of the head and neck. This surgeon has trained four to five years in this field after medical school.

Pediatrician: A physician who has three years of special training in the field of children's medical and surgical problems, after graduating from medical school.

Pulmonologist: An internist who has taken two or three additional years of training to qualify as a specialist in respiratory diseases and critical care medicine.

Sleep disorders specialist: A physician (usually a pulmonologist, neurologist, psychiatrist, or sometimes an otolaryngologist) who has done additional training and obtained experience in this area in order to pass special qualifying examinations for certification by the American Board of Sleep Medicine.

THE NEW FIELD OF SLEEP MEDICINE

Sleep medicine is a relatively new field. REM (rapid eye movement) sleep, for example, was first described in the early 1950s, and the first clinical sleep laboratories were opened in the early 1970s. Some medical schools around the country did not start to include the topics of normal and abnormal sleep in their curriculum until the 1980s. Therefore, many practicing physicians in the community have no knowledge or training in the area of sleep disorders. This is why it is important to understand fully what snoring may represent. Once you understand the signs and symptoms of obstructive sleep apnea, you can select the proper physician to confirm the diagnosis and start effective treatment.

Most diagnoses are made from a personal history of what you have been experiencing. These diagnoses are supported by a physical examination, then confirmed by specific laboratory tests.

NIGHT AND DAY: TAKING YOUR SNORING HISTORY

Snoring and excessive daytime sleepiness are the most common symptoms that bring a person to the attention of a doctor. While some symptoms or problems occur during sleep, other symptoms of sleep apnea are evident during the day. Understanding how sleep-disordered breathing ruins sleep, as discussed in Chapters 1 to 3, will help you realize how such daytime problems as drowsiness, lethargy, and inattentiveness develop.

Nighttime Symptoms

What are some common nighttime findings you may report to your doctor? Check the snoring symptoms listed in Table 5.2 and see if any describe your situation.

Once you have determined your specific symptoms, keep the list close at hand to share with your doctor. There are still some other symptoms that may occur during sleep and can cause you

TABLE 5.2	

Take a Snoring Quiz

☐ My snoring is terribly loud (the roaring freight train).

☐ My snoring is soft and subtle (the purring kitten).

☐ I have a progressive increase in the loudness or intensity of snoring and then normal, quiet breathing until the crescendo snoring starts again.

☐ I have occasional audible snoring, along with periods of breath-holding during sleep, which my bed partner or family member notices.

☐ The depth of my inhalations is very irregular.

☐ I have an increased effort to breathe at the end of these episodes of breath holding.

☐ I have quiet spells interrupted by gasping, snorting, choking, or moving about in the bed.

☐ I have breath-holding spells that are long and frightening to my bed partner, who worries that I may stop breathing altogether.

☐ Sometimes I have exaggerated or unusual movement, ranging from kicking a leg to various arm movements to whole body movements.

☐ My bed partner tells of times in which I seem to be convulsing as I attempt to start breathing again after a long and tight obstructive event.

☐ In some circumstances, I behave as if drunk when I am really half-awake, half-asleep.

....

to complain of a certain type of insomnia. Each abnormal breathing event may be concluded by an arousal that is long enough or sufficiently intense to awaken you. In some cases, you may sense a full urinary bladder and then get up to go to the bathroom. If the breathing problem had not occurred, you would have slept through the night and emptied your bladder in the morning. You might then have been concerned that your nighttime awakenings were caused by a urological problem and seen a urologist if the awakenings were frequent. Or, you may see a psychiatrist or family physician for this sleep problem, known technically as a *disorder of maintaining sleep*.

Daytime Sleepiness

The main daytime symptom from snoring or sleep apnea is excessive sleepiness. It is important to note that with pure snoring or snoring not associated with obstructive sleep apnea there may be no daytime dysfunction or sleepiness. Nonetheless, in some people who suffer from obstructive sleep apnea, this daytime sleepiness may be very serious. They may not even be aware of how it impacts on their daytime functioning and may even experience brief lapses while at work. One example is when a person misses certain requirements or specifications demanded by a customer because of brief sleep episodes known as *microsleeps*. Sometimes an individual may fall asleep in conferences or business meetings or during sermons or lectures. People with significant sleep apnea may not have seen the end of a movie or a ball game in years.

The most dramatic examples of excessive daytime sleepiness are industrial accidents or motor-vehicle accidents. Various studies have shown that patients with sleep apnea have high accident rates, and many car crashes are attributable to a decreased alertness caused by sleep deprivation as a result of the deranged sleep of sleep apnea sufferers. Interestingly, in just one study of more than 900 adults, ages thirty to sixty, men with five or more apneas and hypopneas (see page 32) per hour of sleep were three times as likely to have at least one car accident in five years than were those without sleep-disordered breathing. Men and women combined who had more than fifteen apneas or hypopneas per hour of sleep had seven times the likelihood of having at least one accident in five years, compared with those without sleep-related breathing problems. Some drivers with sleep apnea who undergo performance testing perform as poorly as those with blood alcohol levels above the legal limit. After treatment of the sleep apnea, the performance improves.

Besides excessive daytime sleepiness, other symptoms may annoy sleep apnea sufferers during their daily activities. Take the Sleepiness Quiz (see Table 5.3) and mark those symptoms that describe your situation.

LOOKING AT THE SNORER: THE PHYSICAL EXAMINATION

If you've had a thorough annual medical checkup, you know that it requires the physician to look you over from head to toe. Various parts of your body must be palpated or touched while others need to be listened to with a stethoscope. If you go to the doctor with

TABLE 5.3	

Sleepiness Quiz

- ☐ I have a headache in the morning upon getting out of bed.
- ☐ I feel scattered aches and pains throughout my body upon arising.
- ☐ I feel fatigue or tiredness that does not go away even after several large cups of strongly caffeinated coffee.
- ☐ I feel in a low mood that does not lift even as I get on with my daily activities.
- ☐ I have felt depressed enough to seek psychiatric help or to obtain antidepressant medications.
- ☐ I feel irritable, impatient, and moody.
- ☐ I often have an inability to maintain social harmony with family and friends.
- ☐ I have trouble learning new information or grasping new ideas.
- ☐ I am unable to recall useful information.

some symptoms suggesting sleep-disordered breathing, the doctor will then focus on certain parts of the physical examination.

Whether or not you are overweight is usually discernible at first sight, but accurate measurement of height and weight is as essential as accurate determination of the vital signs such as blood pressure, heart rate and rhythm, and respiratory rate. The doctor may calculate a body mass index (see page 58) and measure the circumference of your neck or ask about your collar size. The body mass index is your weight in kilograms divided by your height in meters squared. This will give a measure of whether you are overweight or have a risk factor for a serious disease such as OSA.

The doctor will use an understanding of the structural layout of the entrance to the respiratory system and how it works to help determine whether and why you may be experiencing snoring or sleep apnea. (The anatomy of the upper airway and how normal breathing takes place are described in Chapter 1. Abnormalities in the anatomy and function of the gateway to the lungs that predispose to narrowing of the upper airway with resultant snoring or sleep apnea are discussed in Chapter 2.)

The doctor must pay particular attention to the entrance to your respiratory system, including your nose, mouth, and throat, with careful inspection of the nostrils and nasal passages. If you have been complaining of headaches, the doctor may press his or her fingers over the various facial sinuses to find out if there is any tenderness suggesting infection. When the doctor asks you to open your mouth wide and say "Ah," he or she will use a flat wooden stick to push the tongue down to get a good look at the soft palate, uvula, and throat. The soft palate is the structure that makes up the roof of the mouth toward the entrance of the throat. The uvula is that long dangling structure in the back of the throat, and the tonsils are located at either side of the entrance to the throat.

In some people, the tongue is enlarged or positioned far backward, making it difficult to see the other structures. In such people, the size and position of the tongue may be contributing to a sleep-related breathing disorder. The soft palate may hang down to decrease the size of the opening of the back of the throat. The uvula may be elongated, thickened, or swollen because of the battering it undergoes from an intermittent flapping back and forth during snoring. The tonsils may be enlarged; in fact, sometimes they can be so big as to meet in the midline, a state referred to as *kissing*. (Chapter 8 includes more information on the upper-airway examination and gives the surgical approach to snoring and sleep apnea.)

The doctor will look at your facial silhouette from the side to see the shape, size, and position of the mandible. A short jawbone or mandible that is displaced backward is shown in Figure 5.1. This produces narrowing of the airway space at the base of the tongue. You may be asked to grit your teeth or relax your lips to see if there is an *overbite*, a condition defined by when the upper teeth in the front of the mouth overhang the lower teeth by more than three millimeters. An overbite suggests that the jawbone is small or placed in such a position as to cause encroachment of the tongue on the upper airway (see Figure 5.1.)

Using a stethoscope, the doctor will listen at the Adam's apple in the front of your neck when you are inhaling forcefully, to detect telltale noises of pharyngeal or laryngeal constriction. Sometimes these sounds are audible to a bed partner when the sufferer is asleep.

Of course, it is important for the physician to perform a complete physical examination to evaluate your health fully. Occasionally, obstructive sleep apnea is so severe with prolonged episodes of low oxygen levels in the blood that the heart muscle may become damaged. In these circumstances, there may be signs of fluid retention in the lungs or more likely in the feet or ankles. Puffiness (edema) of the feet or ankles may be seen or felt by the doctor. Sometimes you may complain that your shoes are too tight or no longer fit because of prominent swelling.

Occasionally, the doctor may suspect that an overweight person has *hypothyroidism*, a condition in which the thyroid gland puts out subnormal amounts of thyroid hormone. In cases such as this, the doctor may request specific blood tests.

When symptoms and physical signs indicate that you may

FIGURE 5.1

OVERBITE AND A SHORT MANDIBLE ARE
ASSOCIATED WITH OBSTRUCTIVE SLEEP APNEA

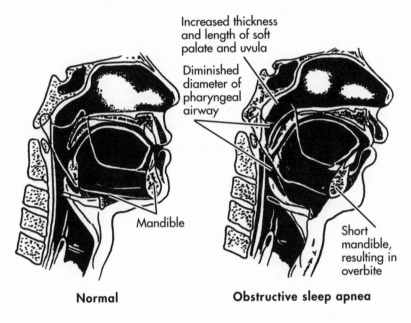

Increased thickness
and length of soft
palate and uvula

Diminished
diameter of
pharyngeal
airway

Mandible

Short
mandible,
resulting in
overbite

Normal

Obstructive sleep apnea

have sleep apnea, a confirmatory sleep study is required. You may want to review these signs and symptoms, which are found in Tables 3.1 and 3.2.

THE EPWORTH SLEEPINESS SCALE

During the physical examination, the doctor may give you a simple questionnaire known as the *Epworth Sleepiness Scale*. This is used by sleep medicine experts for evaluating the tendency to doze during the day. Developed by Dr. Murray Johns, the Epworth Sleepiness Scale (see Table 5.4) involves assigning a number to the likelihood of falling asleep in certain circumstances. To complete the Epworth Sleepiness Scale, determine how likely you are to doze off or fall asleep, as opposed to just feeling tired, during the situations listed in Table 5.4. Consider your usual way of life in recent times. Even if you have not done some of these things recently, try to imagine how they would affect you. Then use the scale provided to choose the most appropriate number for each item. A total score above seven is considered abnormal, and the higher the score, the more likely you will doze off.

TABLE 5.4	

Epworth Sleepiness Scale

SITUATION	CHANCE OF DOZING
Sitting and reading	2
Watching television	1
Sitting, inactive in a public place (for example, in a theater or meeting)	3
As a passenger in a car for an hour without a break	3
Lying down to rest in the afternoon	3
Sitting and talking with someone	1
Sitting quietly after lunch without alcohol	0
In a car, while stopped for a few minutes in traffic	1

Would never doze = 0
Slight chance of dozing = 1
Moderate chance of dozing = 2
High chance of dozing = 3

CLINCHING THE DIAGNOSIS: POLYSOMNOGRAPHY

To find out where on the continuum of sleep-disordered breathing your snoring problem lies, polysomnography must be performed. *Polysomnography* is merely a technical term for sleep study, and this is done in a special laboratory.

Polysomnography includes electroencephalography (EEG), electrooculography (EOG), and electromyography (EMG) to assess the actual quality of your sleep. These tests are explained in Table 5.5 and provide important data that define the time it takes you to fall asleep, the duration of your sleep, and the time you spend in the different stages of sleep. Brief arousals, full awakenings, and movements are recorded to determine the severity of the fragmentation of sleep, which might account for daytime sleepiness and other symptoms.

Besides the recording of brain waves, eye movements, and muscle tension, other measurements related to the function of the respiratory system are recorded. These include airflow at the nose and mouth, chest wall and abdominal movements, and blood oxygen levels. To complete the sleep study, leg movements are monitored, and the heart rate and rhythm are recorded by electrocardiography.

Because polysomnography is only concerned with sleep, it is usually done at night, unless you are a shift worker and sleep during the daytime hours. A specially trained technologist will apply several small metal contacts called *electrodes* on your scalp, using a sticky paste. These electrodes will record your brain waves for the EEG. Similar electrodes are placed on your forehead near your eyes, to record eye movements for the EOG. Electrodes are also placed under your chin and on the front of both legs below the knee to record muscle tension and movements on the EMG.

The technician will place special belts around the chest wall and abdomen to register movements corresponding to respiratory efforts, while tiny tubes are placed just below the nose and in front of the mouth to monitor airflow. Electrodes are also placed on the front of your chest to record the electrocardiogram. Finally, a special probe is worn on your finger to measure the level of blood oxygen. All these devices are attached by thin, colorful wires to a small box at the head of the bed, which in turn is attached to the polysomnograph or computer.

It is important to realize that none of these "attachments" are painful, and the whole setup is relatively comfortable. Most people who are selected to be evaluated in the sleep lab can fall asleep without too much difficulty, even though they are attached to so many pieces of equipment. A technician is always nearby to handle any problems during the sleep study. Usually video monitoring is done for safety and to record any unusual movements that may occur during your sleep. All the information is continuously recorded on large, long sheets of paper, or, as is more commonly done today, on computers. In the morning, you will awaken, the

TABLE 5.5	

Polysomnography Tests

Electroencephalography uses an apparatus for recording electrical activity from the brain. Special electrodes or probes are placed on the scalp and attached by wires to an amplifier that can convert the electrical signals to wave-like written forms on papers or as images on a computer screen.

Electrooculography records the electrical voltage that exists between the front and back of the eye. This electrical activity changes along with eye movement and is detected by electrodes placed on the skin near the eye. Movements of the eye will appear as tracings on paper or a screen.

Electromyography involves an instrument that converts electrical activity associated with functioning muscle into a written or visual record. Higher muscle tension will appear as a thicker line on this recording.

devices will be carefully removed, and you will go home. The test is completed.

All of the tracings from the EEG, EOG, EMG, and the respiratory monitors are carefully reviewed, literally second by second, by a trained technologist and a specialized physician. These tracings will help the doctor determine the quality and quantity of sleep, the continuity of airflow at the nose and mouth, and the movements of the abdomen and chest wall. The number of minutes of sleep is counted and the percentage of time spent in each stage is calculated. These specialists count every arousal, awakening, and movement, along with every apnea and hypopnea. The amount of time spent at various oxygen levels is also determined.

SPECIFIC DIAGNOSIS LEADS
TO PROPER TREATMENT

From this kind of sleep study, the nature and severity of your sleep-related breathing disorder can be determined. Importantly, other problems affecting your sleep can also be identified. One such problem may be *nocturnal myoclonus* (*myo* means "muscle," *clonus* means "twitching"), which involves intermittent, periodic movements such as kicking a leg. Each time this movement occurs, it may be associated with a brief arousal from sleep. These periodic limb movements during sleep may also cause symptoms similar to obstructive sleep apnea such as excessive daytime sleepiness or disrupted sleep. Specific medications may help relieve this problem.

Getting a good night's sleep again depends on an accurate diagnosis. Once it is determined that you have "pure" snoring or obstructive sleep apnea, your doctor can prescribe a treatment regimen that can finally relieve and prevent further problems.

CHAPTER 6

Step 2: Maintain a Normal Weight

ell me more about the risk factor I can change, starting today," requested Pete, a successful banker, when he came to the Cleveland Clinic for help in stopping snoring. This once-athletic man had just turned forty and was at least that many pounds over a healthy weight for his height and build. While Pete had snored for years, in the past few months his snoring had worsened. With his wife jabbing his ribs throughout the night to awaken him and stop the snoring, Pete felt tired and lethargic the next day.

As the physician explained to Pete, while there are many ways to cure snoring and obstructive sleep apnea, both surgically and nonsurgically, losing weight is often the best way to guarantee that the cure will work.

SNORING IS A "WEIGHTY" ISSUE

Snoring combined with obesity or obstructive sleep apnea becomes a dangerous issue. It only takes a quick glance in the mirror to know if you would benefit from losing a few pounds. Men may not even need to look into a mirror, as some experts believe an expanding neck measurement says it all, especially for those who have fat stores around their neck. If you are male and your neck is size 17 or larger and has increased over the years, chances are your girth has increased too, adding to your problem with snoring.

Obesity is defined as being 20 percent or more over normal body weight, and it affects one-third of the U.S. population. However, even being slightly overweight can contribute to a snoring problem. Whether you are obese or just carrying around some baby fat, you have great company. According to a Louis Harris and Associates survey in 1997, Americans are fatter than ever before. Seventy-four percent of Americans who are twenty-five years or older are overweight, up from 71 percent in 1996, 69 percent in 1994, 66 percent in 1992, and only 59 percent ten years ago.

Not only does carrying around extra baggage increase your snoring, weighing as little as ten or fifteen pounds over your desired weight can exacerbate a heart condition, elevate blood pressure and cholesterol levels, and even increase your risk of certain cancers. In the midst of the pessimistic outlook for overweight individuals, there is some good news. While gaining weight can increase the chance of snoring, as well as serious illness, losing weight can reduce the risk.

OBESE OR PLEASINGLY PLUMP?

"Then how much should I weigh? I have to starve to weigh what the doctor's height/weight chart says." While height and weight charts used to give an accurate range, newer studies show that your body mass index (BMI) gives a more accurate picture of health. BMI is defined as body weight (in kilograms) divided by height (in meters squared). The BMI number or value correlates to a risk of adverse effects on health, with higher numbers showing an increased risk. According to the American Dietetic Association, people with a higher percentage of body fat tend to have a higher BMI than do those who have a greater percentage of muscle. It is this extra body fat, not muscle, that puts you at greater risk for health problems.

Using the BMI chart (Figure 6.1), locate the height closest to your height along the left hand column. Then starting at that number, run your finger across the horizontal line until you find the weight closest to your weight. Now go up the column to find your BMI. For example, if you weigh 180 pounds and are five feet, eight inches tall, your BMI according to this chart is 27. Based on Table 6.1, a BMI of 27 puts you at low risk for health problems related to body weight.

BALANCING CALORIES AND ACTIVITY

It is important to understand that each person is different. While your colleague may be the same height as you yet weigh twenty pounds less, both of you may be at your optimal weight, depending on certain variables. These variables include not only your height, but also your age, bone structure, and genetics.

"OK. Bring out the lettuce. I guess it's time to get back on a diet." Shelly vowed to do anything possible to put an end to her nighttime snoring. Not only was it disrupting her sleep, making it difficult to stay awake or concentrate at work, but also her husband slept in the guest bedroom on the other side of their home.

The truth is, in the past five years, comprehensive scientific studies have shed light on the impact of deprivation diets on weight loss, and the findings have consistently held true: Diets alone do *not* work. In fact, if anything, dieting only makes you gain weight by training your body to store fat rather than burn it. Yes, deprivation dieting can help you lose weight. Yet for most people who eat less, one-third of this loss is a reduction of muscle—not fat—and lean muscle (as opposed to body fat) is what helps burn calories.

Scientific studies show that *fat burns two to three calories per pound* while *muscle burns fifty calories per pound*. Muscle mass is metabolically active tissue, meaning that it is the tissue that burns calories.

FIGURE 6.1
BODY MASS INDEX (BMI)

Height (inches)	19	20	21	22	23	24	25	26	27	28	29	30	31	32	33	34	35
58	91	96	100	105	110	115	119	124	129	134	138	143	148	153	158	162	167
59	94	99	104	109	114	119	124	128	133	138	143	148	153	158	163	168	173
60	97	102	107	112	118	123	128	133	138	143	148	153	158	163	168	174	179
61	100	106	111	116	122	127	132	137	143	148	153	158	164	169	174	180	185
62	104	109	115	120	126	131	136	142	147	153	158	164	169	175	180	186	191
63	107	113	118	124	130	135	141	146	152	158	163	169	175	180	186	191	197
64	110	116	122	128	134	140	145	151	157	163	169	174	180	186	192	197	204
65	114	120	126	132	138	144	150	156	162	168	174	180	186	192	198	204	210
66	118	124	130	136	142	148	155	161	167	173	179	186	192	198	204	210	216
67	121	127	134	140	146	153	159	166	172	178	185	191	198	204	211	217	223
68	125	131	138	144	151	158	164	171	177	184	190	197	203	209	216	223	230
69	128	135	142	149	155	162	169	176	182	189	196	203	209	216	223	230	236
70	132	139	146	153	160	167	174	181	188	195	202	209	216	222	229	236	243
71	136	143	150	157	165	172	179	186	193	200	208	215	222	229	236	243	250
72	140	147	154	162	169	177	184	191	199	206	213	221	228	235	242	250	258
73	144	151	159	166	174	182	189	197	204	212	219	227	235	242	250	257	265
74	148	155	163	171	179	186	194	202	210	218	225	233	241	249	256	264	272
75	152	160	168	176	184	192	200	208	216	224	232	240	248	256	264	272	279
76	156	164	172	180	189	197	205	213	221	230	238	246	254	263	271	279	287

Body Weight (pounds)

TABLE 6.1	

Body Mass Index

BMI	RISK FOR HEALTH PROBLEMS RELATED TO BODY WEIGHT
20–25	Very low risk
26–30	Low risk
31–35	Moderate risk
36–40	High risk
40+	Very high risk

The more muscle mass your body has, the more calories you burn all day, even while you are sitting around.

Studies show that approximately 95 percent of people who go on weight-loss diets will gain all or some of it back within one year. In fact, some studies found that after a period of five years, not one "advertised" diet program was successful in keeping the weight off.

The best way to maintain or reach an ideal weight is to burn more calories than you take in, through exercise and activity. A problem that obese people are confronted with is that many underestimate how much they really eat, and they may actually need to increase their amount of exercise more than slightly over-weight adults need to, in order to burn enough calories for weight loss. This problem with energy consumption may continue even after the obese person gets closer to a normal weight. Nutritionists conclude that among those who are successful at keeping off the weight, more than 95 percent are exercisers—and most are walk-ers. So, while you are busy figuring out how many calories you need to burn to lose extra pounds, let's go ahead and talk about another painful issue: moving around more.

YOUR SNORING TREATMENT: EXERCISE
···

If you dread the thought of working out, or the word *exercise* makes you run—the other way—keep reading. Government statistics show that 60 percent of all Americans do not get regular exercise, a statistic that has remained steady in the last two decades. Isn't it ironic that each year the American public spends $30 billion on diet foods and diet programs while exercise costs nothing and is the key to maintaining a normal weight?

"I used to exercise, but now my knees hurt from arthritis, and sometimes it is all I can do to get to work each day." Jake, a sixty-three-year-old attorney, was painfully honest about how aging joints and a tired body had tainted his relationship with exercise. Most of us do slow down with age. According to the Centers for Disease Control and Prevention, 56 percent of men and 44 percent of women between ages eighteen and twenty-nine exercise regularly. These numbers drop to 44 percent and 40 percent, respectively, among people thirty to forty-four years old.

Nonetheless, exercise or simply moving around more with exercise will help you lose weight, and that will decrease your snoring. When you stop snoring, erratic sleep symptoms will ease, and you will have the energy to move around even *more*. The vicious cycle of snoring can be stopped by changing bad habits.

CHANGING A LIFETIME OF BAD HABITS
···

For those who suffer from years of starvation diets and weight cycling—up ten pounds, then down fifteen, then up twenty, and down ten—*there is hope, if you are committed to changing bad habits.* Recent findings suggest that some lifestyle changes can lead to successful long-term weight management. These changes include the following:

• Adopt a low-fat diet.

• Begin an exercise program for life.

- Find social support for these lifestyle changes.

- Accept yourself at your healthiest weight, even though it may not be your thinnest.

- Stop the cycle of losing weight only to regain it.

Changing a lifetime of poor eating habits is *not going to be easy*. While there are no shortcuts to losing weight, the bottom line is that you must expend more calories than you take in. To be successful at weight reduction, you will need to stay motivated *even when you don't feel like it*.

THE SEVEN SNORING-CURE WEIGHT LOSS HABITS

Look at the following seven snoring-cure weight loss habits and try to adopt these in your daily life.

Habit 1: Stop Deprivation Dieting, and Eat for Good Health

Now that you know that deprivation or fad diets don't work, you can lean on research from the experts. The National Institutes of Health (NIH) revealed that true weight-loss success can happen only if you change your eating habits for good—for a lifetime. You already have certain habits such as brushing your teeth that you do without thinking twice. Eating a low-fat, healthy diet must also become a natural part of your daily life—a true eating habit change that will result in weight loss.

The Food Guide Pyramid (see Figure 6.2) from the U.S. Department of Agriculture (USDA) provides an illustration of how you should eat to stay lean and healthy. It recommends plenty of low-fat, nutrient-dense foods such as fruits, vegetables, cereal, bread, and pasta, with less of an emphasis on whole milk products and high-fat meats. The foundation of the diet, like the pyramid, should be built on the plant foods—fruits, vegetables, and grain products. That does not mean you have to eliminate the milk and

FIGURE 6.2

FOOD GUIDE PYRAMID

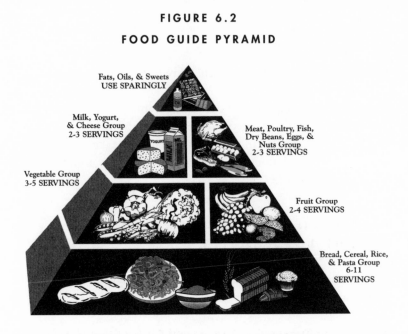

meat or meat-substitute groups. You can use low-fat versions of these foods to complement the rest of the plant-based diet. Fats and sweets should be used sparingly, especially in people trying to lose weight, as they contribute extra calories but few nutrients.

The placement of the beans and peas in the Food Guide Pyramid can be misleading. They are found in the meat and meat-substitute group, which may indicate to you that they should be limited. This is quite the contrary. Beans and peas are low in fat and high in complex carbohydrates; therefore, they *should not be limited* as high-fat meats should be. Beans and peas provide a protein similar to other proteins in this group and make a great meat substitute.

Choosing from the Food Guide Pyramid

In using the Food Guide Pyramid, be sure to follow these guidelines:

- Choose more servings from the plant groups (bread, cereal, rice, pasta, fruit and vegetable).

- Choose fewer servings from animal groups (milk, meat).

- Choose fats and sweets sparingly, especially for weight reduction.

What Is Your Eating Style?

If any single diet program or eating style worked for everyone, we would all be thin. As you may have noticed, we're not. So, what may help you reduce to a normal weight might not work for your friend or colleague. Because we are all different, some people like to have a specific food plan to follow as they initiate healthy lifestyle changes, while others would rather have the freedom to select foods that appeal to them.

Some very-low-calorie diets, high-protein diets, and liquid diets are useful in clinical settings, *but* you need professional supervision and monitoring to participate in these safely. Some popular eating "plans" are very healthy and can help you lose weight. If you wish to use one of the described plans, check with your doctor or certified nutritionist to make sure that all your nutritional needs are met.

Here are two of the best ones:

- **Low-fat diet.** A very-low-fat diet appears to work for those seriously ill with heart disease, as Dr. Dean Ornish described in his book *Eat More, Weigh Less* (HarperCollins, 1993). This heart-healthy diet includes mostly carbohydrates, some protein, and very little fat (less than 10 percent). Although it was formulated to heal ailing hearts, it is also helpful for cancer prevention and weight loss. Before you start piling on the fruits and vegetables, you must know that the only way you can cut fat to 10 percent of calories is to eliminate more sources of animal protein from your diet. Check with your doctor to see if this would benefit you.

- **The vegetarian diet.** Some people believe that vegetarianism is the "new wave" of medicine for the future as plants have many benefits in the prevention of chronic diseases and obesity. A vegetarian diet centers around high-fiber and low-fat meals consisting of fruits, vegetables, whole grains, nuts, and seeds. While 14 million Americans claim to be strict vegetarians, more than 46 percent or 120 million Americans are reducing meat consumption. Review the terms in Table 6.2 to see which type of vegetarianism appeals to you.

Habit 2: Watch Your Portions

No matter what eating plan you decide upon, portion sizes can make or break a weight-reduction program. You can be on target with the right foods for weight reduction but if you eat too much of these foods, you have sabotaged your goal of losing weight. An understanding of portion size is crucial to significantly reducing your weight. Table 6.3 indicates just how much a serving is in the Food Guide Pyramid.

Habit 3: Check the Lowdown on Fat

While researchers used to believe that counting grams of fat would allow you to lose weight, we now know this is not always the case.

TABLE 6.2	

What Type of Vegetarian Are You?

Quasi-vegetarian: You can eat plants and fish and poultry but not red meat.
Pescatarian: You can eat plants and fish.
Lactovegetarian: You can eat plants and dairy products.
Lacto-ovovegetarian: You can eat plants, dairy products, and eggs.
Ovovegetarian: You can eat plants and eggs.
Vegan: You can eat a strict plant-based diet with no animal by-products such as milk or honey.

It is true that because fat is calorie dense and provides nine calories per gram, limiting foods loaded with fat automatically limits your calorie intake, leading to weight loss. Carbohydrate and pro-

TABLE 6.3	

Serving Sizes According to the Food Guide Pyramid

Bread, Cereal, Rice, and Pasta

1 slice of bread
1/2 hamburger bun (1 bun would equal two bread servings)
1/2 bagel (1 whole bagel would equal two bread servings)
1/2 English muffin
3/4 ounce of pretzels
1/2 cup of cooked cereal, pasta, and rice
1 ounce of cold cereal

Fruit

1 medium piece of fruit
1/2 cup of chopped, cooked, or canned fruit
1/2 cup of fruit juice

Vegetables

1/2 cup cooked
1 cup raw

Milk

1 cup of nonfat milk
1 cup of nonfat, sugar-free yogurt
1 1/2 ounces of fat-free cheese

Meat and Meat Substitutes

2 to 3 ounces of lean meat, fish, or poultry without the skin
1 cup to 1 1/2 cups of cooked beans
2 eggs or 1/2 cup of low-cholesterol egg alternative

tein, on the other hand, provide less than half the calories of fat, or about four calories per gram. Nonetheless, it must be kept in mind that eating as much low-fat or no-fat foods as you want is not the answer to weight loss. If you eat more calories than you burn off, you will gain weight.

Most Americans consume a diet with 35 to 40 percent of the calories from fat. The American Heart Association, the American Cancer Society, and the National Academy of Sciences all recommend that Americans reduce their fat calories to less than 30 percent of total calories. Some researchers recommend trying to keep fat calories to less than 20 percent, although that is not always easy. Unfortunately, fatty foods usually taste better, and that adds to this "weighty" challenge. Tasty substitutes have to be enjoyed sometimes or you will find yourself bingeing (overeating) on high-fat, high-calorie foods. For example, you might eat a favorite low-fat frozen yogurt instead of ice cream, or barbecued chicken instead of a fatty steak.

As you reduce the fat in your diet, seek balance. Each individual food does not have to have 20 to 30 percent of the calories or less as fat. Remember, fruits and vegetables have little or no fat, while some foods such as low-fat cheese may have 50 percent of the calories as fat. The idea is to balance high- and low-fat foods over the course of the day and week.

While you are watching the fat content of your diet, perhaps the most important fats to stay away from are saturated fats and trans fatty acids. A diet high in *saturated fat* (the type of fat in meat and dairy products) and *trans fatty acids* (the type of fat in margarine, snack and fast-food products, crackers, pastries, and many processed foods) can lead to many types of cancer, obesity, and heart disease.

Read the Label

To determine whether a food is high, moderate, or low in fat, as well as what type of fat it has, it is important to read the label. Package labels include the ingredients, the calories, the fat content, the nutrients, the sodium and fiber content, and much more for the consumer's information (see sample label in Table 6.4). After reading the label, you can figure out the fat content of favorite foods by using the formula in Table 6.5. Table 6.6 defines some of the terms used on product labels, and Table 6.7 provides a list of low-fat alternatives for your diet.

TABLE 6.4

Sample Label
Kraft Natural Finely Shredded Parmesan Cheese

Ingredients: Part-skim milk, cheese culture, salt, enzymes, aged over 10 months

NUTRITION FACTS

Serving size 2 Tsp (5g)
Servings per container 17

Amount Per Serving

Calories 20
Calories from Fat 10

% DAILY VALUE*

Total Fat 1.5g	2%
Saturated Fat 1g	5%
Cholesterol less than 5mg	1%
Sodium 75mg	3%
Total Carbohydrate 0g	0%
Dietary Fiber 0g	0%
Sugars 0g	
Protein 2g	
Vitamin A 0%	Vitamin C 0%
Calcium 4%	Iron 0%

*Percent Daily Values are based on a 2,000-calorie diet. Your daily values may be higher or lower depending on your calorie needs.

Habit 4: Don't Forget That Calories Do Count

Not surprisingly, even with all the media hype about eating "low-fat" foods to lose weight, researchers have taken an about-face, now saying that calories still count. The American Dietetic Association recommends a calorie level of *no less than ten times your desired weight*, with women getting at least 1,200 calories and men getting at least 1,400 calories per day. This is good news for those dieters who have tried to maintain very-low-calorie diets with little success. For example, if your goal is 130 pounds, you should eat

TABLE 6.5	

High or Low Fat?

1 gram of fat = 9 calories.
If the serving has 2 grams of fat, then
2 × 9 = 18 calories from fat.
If the total number of calories for a serving are 100, then
18/100 = 18% of calories from fat.

TABLE 6.6	

Labels Can Be Confusing

Low-fat means a product has no more than 3 grams of fat per serving.
Low saturated fat means it has no more than 1 gram of saturated fat per serving.
Reduced fat means the product has at least 25 percent less fat per serving than the traditional item.
Light means the product has one-half the fat or one-third the calories of its regular counterpart.
Fat-free has ½ gram of fat or less per serving.

TABLE 6.7	

Get the Fat Out

If you find it difficult to achieve the goal of consuming less than 20 or 30 percent of your calories from fat, try these low-fat alternatives in your diet:

INSTEAD OF	TRY
Butter, margarine	Fat-free spreads and sprays (few calories) and reduced-sugar jams, jellies, and preserves
Whole milk	1% or skim milk
Cheeses	Fat-free or low-fat cheeses, part-skim milk cheeses
Snack crackers, chips, microwave popcorn	Pretzels, rice cakes, Melba toast, air-popped popcorn or reduced-fat microwave popcorn, raw vegetables
Baked goods, cookies	Fresh or canned fruit, graham crackers, vanilla wafers, gingersnaps, angel food cake, animal crackers
Frozen ice cream bar	Fruit juice popsicle, frozen fruit and juice popsicle, sorbet, frozen ice-milk fudge bar
Fried foods	Baked, grilled, broiled, steamed, roasted, or microwaved foods; use nonstick spray to saute
Salad dressings	Fat-free salad dressings
Sour cream	Fat-free sour cream
Cream cheese	Fat-free cream cheese
Whole-milk yogurt	Low-fat or nonfat yogurt

around 1,300 calories per day. If your goal is 180 pounds, then you can follow a diet of 1,800 calories per day for weight reduction. This daily calorie allowance will not allow a quick reduction of weight, but studies show that it is better to make lifestyle changes and lose weight slowly in order to keep it off for good.

Habit 5: Eat Frequently

It is interesting that when most of us decide to lose weight, we immediately stop eating. Researchers now know that the best way to maintain a normal weight is to stop dieting, and to eat more frequently with minimeals. Dieting can often be hazardous to your health as it restricts calories and nutritious foods, causing you to feel depressed and deprived, resulting in rebound bingeing or overeating. Contrary to deprivation dieting, eating *more frequently* will boost your metabolism and productivity. Research has found that people who eat two meals or less during the day have a slower metabolic rate (the speed at which your body burns calories, and the rate that we all want to go faster) versus those who eat three or more times a day. Eating frequently will also keep your blood glucose constant so you do not feel irritable or overly hungry.

An easy way to adjust to minimeals is to break your daily food intake into five or six small meals, spaced every three to four hours throughout the day. Each minimeal will have about 200 to 300 calories, depending on your total caloric goal. Your daily menu may look like this:

Minimeal 1: 1 egg, 1 slice of toast, 1 cup of skim milk, coffee

Minimeal 2: 1 cup of plain yogurt, 1 cup of strawberries

Minimeal 3: 3 ounces of water-packed tuna, low-fat mayonnaise, lettuce, tomato, 2 slices of bread, 1 apple, tea

Minimeal 4: 2 graham crackers, 1 tablespoon of peanut butter, ½ cup of skim milk

Minimeal 5: 3 ounces of baked skinless chicken breast, 1 baked potato with low-fat sour cream, 1 cup of steamed broccoli, ½ cup of cooked carrots, mineral water

Minimeal 6: 3 cups of air-popped popcorn, ½ cup of red grapes

Habit 6: Keep a Food Diary

As you start a lifestyle plan to lose weight to help end snoring, keeping a food diary may help you stay on track. Keeping a food diary helps you know exactly where you stand nutritionally. You may think you are eating a healthful diet and watching your portions, but then after calculating your calories at the end of the day, you find that you have eaten twice as many as you thought.

In fact, studies have shown that when obese people who say they maintain a low-fat, low-calorie diet are asked to record their daily food intake, the results are surprising. The same people who said they ate no more than 1,100 calories per day topped off at an average of over 2,000 calories per day. This made a tremendous difference that resulted in weight gain instead of loss!

Until you get in the good health "habit," keeping a food diary will help keep you organized and honest. Use it as you would a checkbook, writing down what you eat each day, the portion size, and the calorie and fat counts. As you go through the day, calculate the calories in your diet. If your calorie intake is over the suggested limits for weight loss, make adjustments the next day. The diary is a good indicator of what you really eat.

Copy the following food diary format (Table 6.8) in a notebook, and use this as motivation to stick with your eating plan for good health. Don't be hard on yourself, but use this as a learning and awareness tool.

Habit 7: Move Around More

No, you do not have to train for a marathon to drop pounds and get to a normal weight. But it might help if you put your exercise commitment in writing—and the exercise does not have to be

TABLE 6.8	

Food Diary (Sample)

DAY	PORTION SIZE	CALORIES AND/OR FAT GRAMS
Minimeal 1	1 small bagel	160 calories
	2 slices low-fat cheese	90 calories
	1 orange	60 calories
Minimeal 2	1 low-fat yogurt	100 calories
Minimeal 3	1 bowl vegetable soup	150 calories
	6 wheat crackers	80 calories
Minimeal 4	2 graham crackers	60 calories
	1 tablespoon peanut-butter	90 calories
	1 cup low-fat milk	90 calories
Minimeal 5	3 ounces chicken breast	120 calories
	Romaine lettuce with nonfat dressing	50 calories
	1 small baked potato	90 calories
	1 cup broccoli	50 calories
Minimeal 6	3 cups popcorn	80 calories

painful. Even though your colleague may thrive on running five miles each day, according to experts from the American College of Sports Medicine (ACSM) and the Centers for Disease Control and Prevention, the "*no pain, no gain*" theory is *out*. These experts say that we should strive to accumulate thirty minutes of moderate-intensity physical activity every day of the week, or enough to burn about 200 calories (equal to a brisk two-mile walk). This exercise can be done all at one time, *or* you may break it into smaller segments, depending on your time and commitment.

Several short sessions of exercise with available home training equipment may be the most effective exercise program for many overweight people. A study by University of Pittsburgh researchers found that those who used home exercise equipment for short "bursts" of exercise throughout the day were most able to stay with a fitness program. You could do ten minutes of aerobic exercise with your video before work, walk on a stair-machine for ten minutes after lunch, take a ten-minute jog on your treadmill before dinner, and then end your day with a ten-minute ride on your stationary bike while watching the news.

If the short bursts of exercise at home appeal to you, consider building your own home gym. Check the classified advertisements for used exercise equipment such as electronic treadmills or stationary bicycles, but be sure to use them for more than hanging clothes at the end of the day.

If you don't want to buy gym equipment, you can get enough exercise to lose weight and stay in shape with walking, swimming, water aerobics, and even heavy yard work or gardening. All of these, if done regularly, will burn the calories.

Look into buying a popular exercise video. There are instructional videos for all levels of fitness. You can get up ten minutes earlier in the morning, pop in the tape, and get moving—no matter how inclement the weather is outside. Yes, there are *no* excuses!

Whether you do it all in one period or break it up throughout your day, for most people, a regular exercise program will help burn fat, reduce weight, and stop snoring. If you didn't change what you ate, yet burned an additional 200 calories a day, you would lose about twenty pounds in one year.

Something for Everyone

So what type of exercise do you enjoy? Table 6.9 shows popular warm–weather exercises and the wintertime equivalents based on the average number of calories burned per hour. Of course, this amount is an estimate and may vary, depending on your weight and how hard you work out (or lay back!).

Use Table 6.10 to choose the activities that are pleasurable and that you will stick with. Depending on your personal fitness level, vary the exercises to keep yourself from getting bored. Doing the same exercise repeatedly is like having peanut butter and jelly sand–

TABLE 6.9

Warm-Weather Sports and Wintertime Equivalents

GO FOR THE BURN	CALORIES PER HOUR	COOL-WEATHER WORKOUTS
Aerobics (low impact)	400	Snow shoveling (light)
Cycling (10 mph)	300	Stationary bike (10 mph)
Gardening	280	Window cleaning
Golf (walking)	300	Splitting logs
Hiking on steep hills	400	Indoor climbing
Mowing a lawn	275	Mopping floors
Rowing	400	Rowing machine
In-line skating	450	Step aerobics
Swimming	400	Skiing (cross country)
Tennis (doubles)	235	Indoor basketball
Tennis (singles)	390	Racquetball
Badminton	250	Indoor volleyball
Walking (3 mph)	250	Mall walking

wiches every day for lunch—it just gets old. As seasons change, don't let inclement weather stop you from continuing your exercise "habit." If you enjoyed walking outside during the summer, consider joining an indoor aerobics class this winter. If you were passionate about beach volleyball, check out your local recreation center for the indoor volleyball schedule. Likewise, if you thrive on swimming at the lake, continue this water sport in an indoor pool.

CONSIDER THE BENEFIT—GOOD SLEEP!

Starting and maintaining a healthy weight-control program may not be easy at first. For some, changing their dietary habits to include more fruits and vegetables is difficult—especially if they survived on a diet of fast food. Others find adding exercise—even just thirty minutes a day—a major stumbling block in an already

TABLE 6.10	

Activities and Exercises to Keep You Healthy

Badminton	Jumping rope	Stationary cycling
Baseball	Karate	Strength training
Basketball	Kick boxing	Swimming
Biking	Low-impact aerobics	Tae kwon do
Bowling	Mall walking	Tai chi
Dancing	Mowing a lawn	Tennis
Gardening	Qigong (or chi gong)	Vacuuming
Golf	Rollerskating	Walking
Handball	Rowing	Washing windows
High-impact aerobics	Running	Water exercises
Hiking	Soccer	Yard work
House cleaning	Softball	Yoga
In-line skating	Stair climbing	

harried life. But studies show that people who focus on gradual lifestyle changes and give themselves credit for making positive moves will stay motivated to continue.

It's up to you! Stopping snoring might involve some drastic lifestyle changes, yet these are changes only you can make. Nonetheless, the rewards of being able to sleep soundly and lead an active, normal life are well worth any sacrifices you will make.

CHAPTER 7

Step 3: Try Nonsurgical Treatments

A t this point in *The Snoring Cure*, you should have a clear-cut idea of the reason (or reasons) why you snore. Fully understanding your problem will help you and your doctor find the most successful treatment, be it surgical or nonsurgical. Yet before you choose any treatment, there are two important questions you and your doctor should consider:

1. Do you have *pure snoring*, or is the snoring just one symptom of obstructive sleep apnea?

2. Is your snoring problem caused by an anatomic abnormality, such as a deviated septum or nasal polyps, that can be corrected easily through surgery? (If so, read Chapter 8 for surgical cures.)

The *first question* usually can be answered once your doctor has examined you and learned about your snoring history (see Chapter 5). You have *pure snoring* if you snore but do *not* have

• Significant reductions in airflow through the back of the throat to the lungs.

- Decreases in oxygen levels in the blood.

- Excessive daytime sleepiness or other symptoms as a result of sleep disruption.

If you have daytime sleepiness or any of the other symptoms of obstructive sleep apnea or its milder variants (see page 30), then it is clear that you have *more* than pure snoring. As explained in Chapter 5, polysomnography, or a sleep study, is necessary to evaluate the nature and severity of your sleep-related breathing problem, especially if the doctor believes you have more than pure snoring based on your symptoms.

The *second question* regarding anatomical abnormalities may be more difficult to answer. You could have more than one structural abnormality causing your snoring problem. Or, it may be impossible for your doctor to be exactly sure what structure in the upper airway is causing the snoring or the obstructive sleep apnea. In either case, a complete evaluation of your upper airway is necessary to determine whether surgery would help your situation.

"But I don't want surgery unless it is absolutely necessary." No one does! That's why for most causes of pure snoring, the following nonsurgical methods are usually recommended as the first approach to treating sleep-related breathing disorders.

NONSURGICAL TREATMENTS
TO END SNORING

Lose Weight

As discussed in Chapter 6, obesity is a common risk factor among people who have snoring or obstructive sleep apnea. Consequently, losing weight is the *only nonsurgical method that may cure snoring and sleep apnea in many patients.* The other nonsurgical methods do not produce a true cure but rather only control symptoms. Losing weight is not easy, but it can be done safely if you follow a balanced program that includes reducing fats and calories, along with increasing exercise and activity. Weight loss is discussed in detail in Chapter 6.

If you need to lose a great amount of weight and already feel defeated, it's important to know that reaching a "normal" weight, although desirable for other health reasons, is not necessary for curing snoring. For some people, a *10 to 20 percent* decrease in body weight is all that is needed to achieve a remarkable decrease in snoring, as well as a beneficial reduction in sleep apnea. The exact reason for the improvement is not known, but it is believed to be related to an improvement in the size and function of the upper airway.

Avoid Alcohol and Certain Drugs

While weight gain is a prime contributor to snoring, alcohol and medications that cause drowsiness or muscle relaxation can also worsen snoring and sleep apnea. These agents reduce the force of the muscles that help to keep your upper airway open. If you are a snorer who has a few drinks in the evening, this could result in significant obstructive sleep apnea and health consequences.

Like alcohol, sleeping pills and tranquilizers also cause muscle relaxation and sleepiness, which can prolong the apneas and result in deeper decreases in oxygen levels.

Reduce Nasal Congestion

Avoiding the various triggers of nasal congestion or alleviating the congestion of allergies or rhinitis frequently helps lessen some cases of snoring or very mild obstructive sleep apnea, such as sleep hypopnea syndrome or upper-airway resistance syndrome (UARS). You can take nasal decongestants orally (pill form) or use as a decongestant spray, which is inhaled in each nostril.

Causes of Inflammation, or Rhinitis

Rhinitis, or inflammation of the linings inside the nose, is an extremely common cause of nasal congestion. In fact, rhinitis is one of the most frequent problems seen by doctors in their offices or clinics. Rhinitis caused by an allergy affects as many as 25 million people in the United States. When it is the result of nonallergic causes, rhinitis affects at least another 5 million Americans. Nonallergic rhinitis can be caused by irritants in air pollution, by cigarette smoke, or by weather changes. Allergic rhinitis is caused by an allergy to a specific substance such as cat hair or pollen. The allergic form is more likely to bother younger people, while the nonallergic type tends to strike later in life.

As explained in Chapter 1, the nose helps prepare the air you breathe for arrival in the lungs. Inside the nose are tubular bones called *turbinates*, which humidify, warm, and filter the air. A mucous membrane that is rich in blood vessels covers these turbinates. These turbinates may shrink and swell and even alternate this process from one side to the other. The symptoms of nasal congestion that you feel occur when they swell.

Certain activities or situations affect the size of the turbinates. For example, lying on your back causes the turbinates on both sides of the nose to swell. If you have nasal congestion, lying on your side may reduce the size. Exposure to cold air or inhaling cool air can also make the turbinates swell. Pregnancy, with its hormonal changes, may cause enlargement of the turbinates, and sometimes women who never snored before may start to snore while pregnant until after they give birth. Similarly, hormonal alterations resulting from changes in a woman's menstrual cycle will cause turbinate swelling and consequent snoring. This occurs particularly right before or during the time of the menstrual period.

If nasal congestion is caused by an allergy, the doctor may refer you to an allergy specialist. Especially if the nasal congestion is seasonal and worsens in the spring or fall or worsens after exposure to potential allergens, an allergy may be the culprit. Itchy eyes and nasal drip may also indicate an allergy. Again, seeing an allergist may be helpful. The factors that affect nasal congestion are summarized in Tables 7.1 and 7.2.

TABLE 7.1	

Factors Affecting Nasal Congestion

FACTOR	CONGESTION	DECONGESTION
Lying on back	+	
Lying on side	+	+
Chilling skin	+	
Warming skin		+
Cigarette smoke	+	
Strong odors	+	
Breathing cold air	+	
Breathing rapidly	+	
Pregnancy	+	
Menstruation	+	
Pain (physical)		+
Exercise		+
Emotions		
Frustration	+	
Fear		+
Anxiety	+	
Sexual stimulation	+	

Solving Nasal Congestion

Nonmedical treatments can help reduce congestion. For example, vigorous exercise will produce decongestion of the nasal passages, as will warming of the skin. A warm towel put on the nose and forehead may provide much-needed relief of nasal congestion.

Many types of medications (see Table 7.3) are also used to treat the specific problems of congestion, drippy nose, or other allergy symptoms. Some medications relieve the symptoms, while others such as mast cell stabilizers actually prevent allergy symptoms altogether.

TABLE 7.2	

Common Allergens, Irritants, and Physical Changes That Cause Rhinitis

Plant pollens
Tree pollens
Molds and mildew
Household dust (dust mites)
Animal dander
Industrial chemicals
Cockroaches
Feathers
Foods (chocolate, shellfish, milk, citrus, eggs, nuts, corn)
Food additives or colorings (sulfites or preservatives)
Medications (aspirin, ibuprofen or related drugs, penicillin, beta-blockers)
Insect stings
Hormones
Smoke
Perfumes or inhalants
Respiratory infections
Gases
Weather changes
Cold air
Exercise

Antihistamines

Whether you should take an antihistamine or decongestant when you have nasal congestion depends on the symptoms and the exact triggers of the nasal problem. Antihistamines prevent the effects of histamine on certain cells in the body. *Histamine* is the chemical released from certain cells in the body after being exposed to an

TABLE 7.3	

Medicines Helpful for Rhinitis

TYPE OF MEDICATION	COMMON USES
Antihistamines	Reduce sneezing and drippiness; may relieve congestion from allergy
Decongestants	Reduce nasal stuffiness or congestion
Anticholinergics	Prevent runny, drippy nose
Mast cell stabilizers (cromolyn sodium)	Prevent nasal congestion before exposure to allergens
Steroids	Prevent all allergy symptoms

allergen. It causes the swelling of the membranes in the nose and increases mucous production. During an allergic reaction, you will have symptoms such as a runny, drippy nose, nasal congestion, itchy eyes, and stuffiness. Whereas older forms of antihistamines enter the brain and cause drowsiness, newer forms do not. For this reason, if you have sleepiness because of obstructive sleep apnea, you need to avoid the older, sedating antihistamines.

There are now at least five nonsedating antihistamines available by prescription in the United States that work to prevent the release of histamine in the body (see Table 7.4). Sedating types are available over the counter in drug stores.

Side Effects of Antihistamines

Sedating antihistamines may cause other problems besides sleepiness. If you take these drugs, you may have decreased reaction time and a hard time paying attention. Other side effects include a dry mouth, an overly dry nose, painful or difficult urination, urinary retention, blurred vision, and constipation.

Nonsedating antihistamines do not cause drowsiness or these other side effects but terfenadine (Seldane) and astemizole

TABLE 7.4	

Antihistamines

GENERIC NAME	BRAND NAME
Nonsedating or mildly sedating	
Terfenadine	Seldane
Astemizole	Hismanal
Loratadine	Claritin
Cetirizine	Zyrtec
Fexofenadine	Allegra
Sedating	
Brompheniramine	Dimetane
Chlorpheniramine	Chlor-trimeton
Diphenhydramine	Benadryl
Tripelennamine	Pyribenzamine
Promethazine	Phenergan
Azatadine	Optimine
Hydroxyzine	Atarax, Vistaril
Clemastine	Tavist
Cyproheptadine	Periactin

(Hismanal) have been associated with abnormal heart rhythms. These two drugs need to be prescribed with particular caution and avoided in people who have liver disease, as well as those with other chronic medical problems. Some nonsedating antihistamines should never be taken if other medicines such as antifungal drugs (ketoconazole or itraconazole) or the antibiotic erythromycin are being used. The other sedating antihistamines do not have these restrictions, and all are available in combination with a decongestant. Because decongestants may raise blood pressure and heart rate, they should be avoided in the elderly or those with hypertension or heart conditions.

Decongestants

Decongestants (see Table 7.5) work by reducing blood flow to the turbinates in the nose, which helps to reduce the swelling. While antihistamines work to stop the mucus in the nose from dripping, decongestants help to open up airways, relieving the congestion. Sometimes decongestants make your nose drip more as the mucus is free to flow.

A decongestant spray applied directly into the nose works rapidly and is more effective than a decongestant taken as a pill. The decongestant sprays should not be used for more than five to seven days because they can produce a "rebound effect." A rebound effect is when ongoing use of the inhaled decongestant causes an irritation or an increase in the swelling of the turbinates. While this swelling wears off when the medication is stopped, it may produce

TABLE 7.5

Decongestants

GENERIC NAME	BRAND NAME
Oral	
Pseudoephedrine	Sudafed
Phenylpropanolamine	
Phenylephrine	
Topical long-acting (8 to 12 hours)	
Oxymetazoline	Afrin
Xylometazoline	Neo-Synephrine 12-hr/maximum, Sinex, Otrivin
Topical short-acting (3 to 8 hours)	
Tetrahydrozoline	
Naphazoline	Privine
Phenylephrine	Vicks, Duration, Neo-Synephrine

a vicious cycle of overuse. In other words, the relief you feel will be short-lived, which makes you use the spray more frequently. If you do use a spray decongestant, try the longer-acting form, and remember to observe the "short-term usage" rule.

Side Effects of Decongestants

Oral decongestants can cause side effects such as tremor, jitters, nervousness, difficulty falling asleep, and difficulty urinating, especially in men with enlarged prostate glands. The topical (spray) decongestants are less likely to cause side effects except the rebound effect. If overused, they may produce nasal septum perforations. Again, people with heart problems or high blood pressure should avoid decongestants altogether.

Anticholinergics

Anticholinergics also relieve nasal congestion and hence may help decrease snoring. This type of medicine is particularly helpful for individuals with a clear, watery discharge (rhinorrhea) from the nose. It may work when the antihistamines or other decongestants do not. The most effective one available today is *ipratropium bromide* (Atrovent), a topical spray that comes in two strengths. [The 0.03 percent preparation is useful for allergic and nonallergic rhinitis when the clear, watery discharge is a prominent problem. The 0.06 percent strength is useful when the common cold (coryza) caused by a virus produces nasal drip.] The most common side effect is irritation or excessive nasal dryness that can lead to nose bleeds.

Cromolyn Sodium

Cromolyn sodium (Nasalcrom) blocks the allergic response to allergens. It prevents mast cells, which are located in the linings of the nose, trachea, and bronchial tubes, from releasing histamine (see page 84). Cromolyn sodium works if you use it *before* exposure and should be taken a week or so before the allergy season begins. The benefit of cromolyn sodium is that there are no side effects.

Steroids

Corticosteroids, which are available by prescription only, are the most effective medications available for the treatment of nasal congestion resulting from allergic or nonallergic causes. Compared to topical or inhaled steroids, oral steroid therapy is more effective and its onset of action is quicker. A seven- to ten-day course of prednisone, an inexpensive but quite potent form of steroid, is frequently useful. The doctor may start you at 30 to 50 milligrams of prednisone per day and taper you off 5 to 10 milligrams every two to three days. This is almost always successful in controlling symptoms. Treatment with inhaled cromolyn or steroids may follow this oral therapy.

Side Effects of Inhaled Steroids

There are now at least six inhaled steroids available by prescription (see Table 7.6). Dexamethasone is the most potent, yet this drug may be absorbed in its active form and produce some serious side effects. The other drugs, however, are less likely to be absorbed and are metabolized or cleared quickly from the bloodstream if absorbed. They produce few if any side effects when taken in recommended doses. Nasal irritation is the most common side effect. Sometimes this is severe enough to produce nasal bleeding. If this happens, stop the medicine immediately. Perforation of the nasal septum can occur, and you need to be aware of this problem.

If you use an inhaled nasal steroid spray, do not spray the medication against your nasal septum. Instead, point the tip of the applicator toward the ear of the side you are spraying. Some of these drugs can be conveniently used once a day, and the best time is about an hour before bedtime.

There are many types of containers for inhaled sprays. Work with the doctor to find the best one for your problem. Usually these sprays can be used for several months without a problem, but some doctors recommend that they be used for only five to fourteen days at a time. When your nasal congestion is relieved, you might stop the spray for awhile before it is needed again for another period of treatment.

TABLE 7.6	

Nasal Steroid Inhalers

GENERIC NAME	BRAND NAME
Dexamethasone	Dexacort
Beclomethasone	Beconase, Vancenase
Budesonide	Rhinocort
Flunisolide	Nasalide, Nasarel
Fluticasone	Flonase
Triamcinolone	Nasacort
Mometasone	Nasonex

Avoiding Allergy Triggers

For some people with nasal congestion caused by allergy, taking control of the environment may make a big difference. In some cases, eliminating environmental triggers may even cure the snoring problem.

Go through your home or office, and discover the problem areas. While environmental triggers vary, common triggers include

Aerosols	Mold and mildew
Chemical fumes	Perfume and scented products
Cigarette smoke	Pet dander
Cockroaches	Pollen
Cold air	Tobacco smoke and wood smoke
Dust	Weather fronts
Fresh paint	Wind
Humid air	

Try to eliminate or avoid any known trigger of allergy. In some cases, an allergist may provide relief using immunotherapy (allergy shots). These allergy shots may help to desensitize you to the allergens that would normally trigger a reaction such as rhinitis.

Nasal Dilators

Various nasal dilators have been tried for years to help relieve obstruction inside the nose. Some of these devices are inserted into the nostrils. Needless to say, these have not been popular because of their discomfort and the high level of maintenance required to keep them clean. An external dilator called Breathe *Right* Nasal Strips has been marketed with some success. These strips are available at most drug and grocery stores and are worn on the outside of the nose. They are designed to slightly open the nose near the tip. When stuck to the skin on the front of the nose, the Breathe *Right* Nasal Strip stabilizes the outer walls of the nasal passages with a springboard action to prevent collapse during inspiration. An increased outer opening of the nose tends to decrease resistance to airflow, which may also result in less mouth breathing.

If your snoring is mainly a result of narrowing of the nasal passages, these strips may reduce or eliminate the snoring. Be patient when using these, as it may take a week or two to get back into the habit of keeping your mouth closed while asleep. Also keep in mind that snoring and airway obstruction during apneas occur *behind the soft palate and tongue.* In these cases, nasal dilators may not be helpful in treating sleep apnea. However, using these nasal strips along with nasal continuous positive airway pressure (CPAP) therapy may be helpful in preventing nasal obstruction (see page 94).

Protriptyline

If you have a very mild version of obstructive sleep apnea that occurs predominantly during REM sleep, a medicine called *protriptyline* (Vivactil) may be helpful. Protriptyline is a tricyclic antidepressant drug that works by increasing the activity of the muscles that keep the upper airway open and by decreasing the amount of REM sleep during which the apneas are more frequent. When higher doses of this medicine are needed, such side effects as dry mouth, urinary hesitancy, constipation, and male sexual dysfunction may become a problem. The side effects go away when the drug is stopped. Your doctor may want to try other antidepressants such as fluoxetine (Prozac), which are helpful in some cases.

Other medicines have been tried for the treatment of snoring and obstructive sleep apnea but none have been proved useful.

Oxygen

Increasing the amount or concentration of oxygen that you breathe during sleep may help but only if you have obstructive sleep apnea. Oxygen can be supplied from tanks. Or the doctor can recommend a more practical method for overnight usage: an electric "concentrator" that takes oxygen out of the room air, which is then inhaled through the nose from tiny prongs at the end of a long thin tube that is connected to the machine. Supplemental oxygen increases the oxygen content in the lungs and blood before each apnea; therefore, it can reduce the drop in blood oxygen levels during closing of the upper airway. The oxygen does not eliminate the apneas, and because the oxygen levels are improved, the apneas may be prolonged since arousal ending each apnea is delayed. You will continue to have interrupted sleep that causes daytime sleepiness.

Extra oxygen added to positive airway therapy (see page 94) may be helpful if you also have significant lung disease and have borderline or low oxygen levels in the blood when you are awake. If you cannot tolerate the other methods of treatment, supplemental oxygen may be helpful to reduce the risk of cardiovascular problems.

Positional Therapy

If you are the target of frequent elbow pokes in the middle of the night from a bed partner, you know how changing position can reduce (or increase) snoring. Chances are you have more severe sleep-disordered breathing when you lie on your back than when you sleep on your sides. This may be because the forces of gravity draw your tongue and palate backward when you are on your back. Most diagnostic sleep laboratories keep track of the number of apneas or hypopneas you have during sleep in various positions.

Positional or postural therapy is most effective if you have pure snoring or very mild obstructive sleep apnea that occurs mainly when you sleep on your back. Years ago, the treatment for snoring was to sew a pine cone to the back of the pajama top to prevent the snorer from lying on his back. As you can imagine, that was a bit uncomfortable and many night shirts, bed sheets, and backs were badly scratched or torn. Today, some specialists recommend sewing a tennis ball or two in a sock to the back of the night shirt in the area between the shoulder blades. This forces the snorer to stay on his side.

While there are few scientific studies to prove the benefit of the "tennis ball" technique, there are some good ways to evaluate its effectiveness. Your bed partner can notice whether or not your snoring is reduced or the apnea spells are eliminated. You might feel better during the day, with less tendency to doze. A simple questionnaire such as the *Epworth Sleepiness Scale* (see page 52) may be used for comparison of your tendency to doze off before and after treatment. In more serious cases, monitoring oxygen levels at home may be helpful to see if this positional therapy works. The results obtained during the diagnostic sleep study in the lab can be compared with the results recorded at home on a portable oximeter. Fewer and milder oxygen drops during sleep represent objective evidence to confirm the subjective reports of the bed partner and the patient.

As with all methods of treating snoring, follow-up is important to determine if the treatment continues to work. If you have more prominent symptoms and documented severe obstructive sleep apnea, you are not a good candidate for positional therapy.

Oral Appliances

Since a large portion of obstruction of the upper airway has been attributed to narrowing of the airway at the back of the tongue, tongue-retaining devices have been designed to pull the tongue forward. One of the first types used suction pressure to hold the tongue in a forward position. This appliance relieved partial or complete obstruction at the base of the tongue. Another device was designed to hold the tongue forward and also pull the mandible forward by hooking on the upper and lower teeth. Appliances that were made to pull the tongue forward have not been very popular because they hurt and are uncomfortable.

After a sleep study determines the severity of the sleep apnea, the doctor may recommend an oral appliance or *mandibular advancement device*. These devices are more popular and useful with people who have mild to moderate obstructive sleep apnea. They may be particularly helpful in reducing snoring in people who snore yet do not have significant sleep apnea.

The mandibular advancement device works by clasping onto the upper and lower teeth and pulling the jaw forward. The distance that the jaw is advanced can be gradually adjusted with some devices. In some cases, your dentist or a specialist, called a *dental prosthetist*, may custom fit the device after a thorough physical examination. Oftentimes special X ray views of the facial bones are required. Sometimes adjusting the device takes a long time and requires a lot of trial and error. A sleep study is needed to document whether a certain amount of advancement is adequate in reducing the sleep apnea.

Side Effects of Oral Appliances

Besides being uncomfortable for some people, the side effects of oral appliances may be excessive salivating; malalignment of the teeth, causing problems with bite; and possible pain or damage to the temporomandibular joint.

Oral devices may be quite helpful, however, for mild to moderate obstructive sleep apnea or pure snoring. They are especially helpful if you do not want to use or cannot tolerate nasal CPAP.

Nasal Continuous Positive Airway Pressure

Nasal CPAP is the treatment of choice for most patients with obstructive sleep apnea. *It is almost 100 percent effective and safe for stopping snoring and obstructive sleep apnea.* When the other therapies are not appropriate, you can generally trust nasal CPAP to work. While nasal CPAP is not invasive, it eliminates snoring and reduces the number of sleep-related breathing problems. By doing so, it decreases fragmented sleep and results in less daytime sleepiness or fatigue and fewer problems with mood and memory.

Remember, when you breathe in, your diaphragm (the main breathing muscle) contracts. The diaphragm pushes down into your abdomen, allowing your chest cavity to expand. This results in lowering the pressure inside to a level below the atmospheric pressure outside the body. The low pressure is transmitted up the conducting airways to the nose and mouth where air is forced in by the higher outside pressure. Can you remember when you used to use a paper straw? Imagine sucking on the straw and the straw collapsing because the pressure inside it is lower than that around it. This is what happens to the upper airway during sleep, because the muscles around the airway relax.

Nasal CPAP maintains a positive pressure inside your airway while you breathe. It acts as a support to prevent further narrowing or collapse of your airway, and it actually increases the size of the airway behind the palate and at the back of your tongue (see Figure 7.1).

Nasal CPAP is applied usually by a custom-made, custom-fit mask that is strapped on the nose. This mask is connected by a swivel and flexible hose to a special pump that quietly provides air under pressure to the nose. Instead of the nasal mask, you may prefer "nasal pillows," which are inserted into your nostrils. In some cases, a chin strap is helpful to keep the mouth closed to reduce loss of pressure. A full-face mask may be necessary in select patients.

Whatever device you use, it is important that it is comfortable and that there are no air leaks from the nose or mouth. Leaks will cause severe drying of the nose or mouth because of the high flow of air. There are many different versions of the nasal mask, each using slightly different designs for shape, fitting, and securing to the nose. A variety of materials are also available to make the mask

FIGURE 7.1
CONTINUOUS POSITIVE AIRWAY PRESSURE (CPAP), DELIVERED BY AN AIRWAY MASK, SERVES AS A PNEUMATIC SPLINT TO PREVENT UPPER-AIRWAY OBSTRUCTION

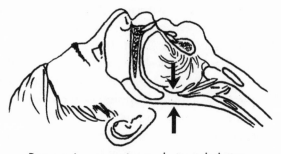

Pressure in upper airway during inhalation
is below atmospheric and may lead to obstruction.

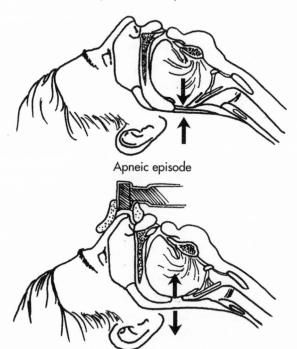

Apneic episode

Nasal CPAP provides pressure above
atmospheric to keep airway open.

comfortable and reduce skin irritations. These materials range from rubbery types, to latex varieties, to the newer "gel" masks, which are particularly soft, form fitting, and comfortable. Sometimes a trial-and-error approach is necessary to find the best mask for you.

While you are asleep in a sleep disorder laboratory, the doctor will be able to find the optimal nasal CPAP level you need to stop the snoring and the other episodes of narrowing in the upper airway. As described in Chapter 5, polysomnography is performed to monitor the airflow at the nose and mouth as well as the movements of the chest wall and abdomen.

The purposes of the first sleep study are to diagnose obstructive sleep apnea and determine its nature and severity. If the doctor decides that nasal CPAP is the best treatment, a second study will be necessary to determine the lowest amount of pressure needed to relieve the decreases in airflow and to maximize the oxygen levels in your blood during sleep. In some cases, split-night polysomnography may be done. This involves being monitored for sleep-related breathing abnormalities during the first part of the night. If significant sleep apnea is found, then during the second part of the night, you will try nasal CPAP to find the right pressure necessary to end the symptoms of obstructive sleep apnea.

During daytime hours at the sleep clinic before the second sleep study is scheduled, or as part of the preparation for a split-night study if that is planned, you will be introduced to the mask and machine. You will try it on and see what it's like breathing with the nasal CPAP machine. If you find the mask reasonably comfortable and your nose has a good airflow, then another night in the sleep laboratory is scheduled. On the second night in the laboratory, all the sleep-stage parameters and respiratory factors including airflow and oxygen levels are monitored. If you understand this process ahead of time, the second night is much more successful. After the required level of nasal CPAP is determined, the doctor will arrange to have the proper mask and machine, set at the appropriate pressure, delivered to your home.

The Challenge

Using nasal CPAP while you are sleeping can be quite a challenge (see Table 7.7). That is why it's important to weigh the inconvenience of the mask against the severity of the snoring or obstructive sleep apnea problem. *It is important to appreciate the potential health-related side effects of untreated sleep apnea (see discussion in Chapter 3).*

To get used to the new equipment, you need to "practice" with the nasal CPAP in the evening while you are awake. Practice can continue for increasingly longer periods of time while you are watching television, reading, or working at a computer. This "desensitization program" will reduce your chances of pulling the mask off during sleep.

Even though nasal CPAP is rarely associated with any serious complications, it may cause you great discomfort, yet most of these obstacles can be remedied. You may have a psychological aversion to the idea of using nasal CPAP every night to sleep, especially if you are newly wed or if you are in a new or developing relationship. Needless to say, a nasal mask may cause you to feel self-conscious. Education regarding obstructive sleep apnea and how treatment is

---

TABLE 7.7	

Obstacles to Nasal Continuous Positive Airway Pressure

Psychological aversion

Claustrophobia

Arousals from sleep

Nasal discomfort, especially dryness

Swallowing air and stomach cramps

Leaks at nose or mouth

Facial skin irritation

Discomfort exhaling

Chest or back pain

beneficial to your optimal health is important to get past this barrier. An understanding and supportive mate is extremely valuable, too.

Claustrophobia can be overcome with some reassurance regarding the safety of nasal CPAP. A desensitization program is also very useful. Tranquilizers that relax the muscles in the upper airway are generally not a good idea. If you find the nasal CPAP mask to be intimidating, you may change to nasal pillows that fit inside the nose.

The most common obstacles to nasal CPAP usage are related to the nose and include drying, irritation, and congestion. To relieve nasal dryness, try using a humidifying system within the nasal CPAP unit itself or a room humidifier placed near the machine. Sometimes nasal drip can be reduced by the normally drying effects of the high airflow from nasal CPAP. Nasal irritation can be reduced by applying a thin film of petroleum jelly or a vitamin A and D ointment to the skin lining the inside of the nostrils. Nasal congestion can be relieved by using an over-the-counter nasal spray such as a 12-hour preparation of xylometazoline (Neo-Synephrine) or oxymetazoline (Afrin). If congestion persists, a nasal steroid spray may be required (see page 89). If you must take a decongestant for rhinitis, use the least amount of medicine required to relieve the congestion.

Other problems you may encounter with the nasal CPAP include swallowing air and skin irritation. You can avoid swallowing air by altering your posture during sleep with various pillows or by changing the type of mask used. Belching or flatulence may be relieved by certain medications such as simethicone. Facial skin irritation can be avoided by carefully selecting the mask and straps that fit your face. Tightening the mask too much can cause damage to the skin. Mouth breathing can be controlled by using a chin strap.

You may find it hard to fall sleep after putting on the nasal CPAP mask because the positive airway pressure feels uncomfortable or is disturbing. You can avoid this by finding a machine with a "ramp" device built into it. This device allows the positive airway pressure to start at a low level (about 5 centimeters of water) and gradually be increased to the full pressure (15 centimeters of water required by prescription to get rid of the apneas). This increase in pressure is achieved over a period of fifteen to forty-five minutes and allows you ample time to drift off to sleep. The higher pressure is then maintained the rest of the night.

In certain cases, you may have trouble exhaling against what seems to be a relatively high positive pressure. This discomfort during exhalation can be solved by a desensitization program as mentioned earlier. Sometimes, it is necessary to switch to the bilevel positive air pressure machine called *BiPAP*. This unit can provide a lower pressure during the expiratory cycle compared with the inspiratory period and will make it easier to exhale. The problem is that the BiPAP machines are about twice as expensive as the regular nasal CPAP devices. In addition, it may be difficult to adjust the BiPAP to the exact levels needed to optimally abolish the apneas and hypopneas. You need to keep in mind that the BiPAP machine may increase your chance of sticking to therapy if you cannot tolerate nasal CPAP.

If you have chest or back pain caused by overinflating or stretching of the chest wall, a slight decrease in the nasal CPAP level or using a BiPAP machine will help to eliminate this.

The newest advance in nasal positive airway pressure therapy is called *auto-CPAP* or *demand-PAP*. The machine automatically adjusts the airway pressure throughout the night according to the breathing patterns of the person using the system. Changes in pressure, up or down, will be based on detection of apneas, snoring, or limitations as airflow is monitored by the machine. This type of device may be appropriate in selected patients with sleep apnea.

STILL NO CURE?

If after trying these nonsurgical methods you are still struggling with the symptoms of a sleep-related breathing problem, there are still some treatment methods that can help. Chapter 8 discusses the best surgical cures and will let you know how each is done, who is a candidate for the various operations, and the effectiveness and side effects of each procedure. Don't give up in your search for the snoring cure. Exhaust all possibilities until you finally achieve the goal of undisturbed, healing sleep.

Step 4: Use the Surgical Snoring Cures

ou've tried the nonsurgical treatments, yet you still can't stop snoring. Don't worry, you are not alone. There are more options to consider, and while the final step—using surgical snoring cures—is more invasive, it does end the problem in most cases.

NEW PROCEDURES TO CURE SNORING

Surgery for snoring dates back to the 1960s when a Japanese physician described a procedure that removed the tonsils and palate, thus decreasing sleep apnea and snoring. Before then, tracheostomy (putting a tube in a small opening in the trachea) was the only procedure available. Since that time, surgeons have extensively studied the problem and have come up with a myriad of successful procedures to decrease or eliminate snoring and sleep apnea.

Before your doctor will perform surgery, a complete evaluation, including a detailed interview and physical examination as described in Chapter 5, will be done to see if you have pure snoring or sleep apnea. If sleep apnea is suspected, a presurgical evaluation, requiring a sleep study or polysomnography, will determine its severity and nature. This evaluation is very important to determine what type and location of anatomic abnormality you may have, as well as the degree of obstructive sleep apnea.

To guarantee surgical success, a critical evaluation of the upper airway by an ear-nose-throat surgeon (ENT or otolaryngologist) is also essential (see page 44). An ENT specialist has trained four to five years in this field after graduating from medical school. The ENT doctor will obtain a thorough history of your symptoms and medical problems, perform a careful physical examination, fiberoptically visualize the upper airway, and sometimes order imaging studies (cephalometrics, computerized tomography, and magnetic resonance imaging) to determine where the obstruction is located. You will probably be awake for these exams.

CORRECT YOUR ANATOMY

Once the surgeon has determined the possible sites causing obstruction and snoring, then the surgical options are explained. Surgery is performed only after the risks and benefits are fully discussed and the medical options described in Chapters 6 and 7 have been tried without success. Since the surgical procedures have formidable names, and the anatomy of the upper airway is complicated, it is important that you ask many questions in order to understand how the operation(s) may help, as well as the possible risk factors.

Depending on the type of obstruction you have, different surgical procedures are used (see Table 8.1). Your surgeon may do these procedures individually, at the same time as other procedures, or sequentially with other operations, depending on your specific anatomic problems.

The procedures described here have been recognized as most successful in curing snoring. Your doctor will decide which one is best for you. It should be emphasized that because of the deranged anatomy and the abnormal function (tendency to collapse or close)

TABLE 8.1	

Surgical Procedures Used to Treat Snoring and Sleep Apnea

Nasal surgery
Septoplasty, turbinate resection
Sinus surgery
Tonsillectomy
Adenoidectomy
Uvulopalatopharyngoplasty (UPPP)
Linguoplasty and glossectomy
Genioglossus advancement with hyoid myotomy (GAHM)
Sliding genioplasty
Laser-assisted uvulopalatoplasty (LAUP)
Radiofrequency tissue volume reduction
Maxillomandibular advancement osteotomy (MMO)
Tracheostomy

of the upper airway, your surgeon and anesthesiologist will take cautionary measures to ensure your safety. Keeping the airway open at the start of anesthesia and upon waking up from the operation may be difficult. Therefore, close monitoring and supervision are essential. Pain medications, tranquilizers, and anesthetics can worsen your obstruction. In fact, you may have a worsening of obstructive sleep apnea in the period shortly after surgery. In many cases, nasal continuous positive airway pressure (CPAP) is used after the operation until the surgical cure is confirmed.

NASAL SURGERY

If you have nasal obstruction and do not breathe well through your nose, you have a higher nasal resistance to airflow, which is even greater during sleep. Numerous studies have shown that nasal obstruction and increased resistance can cause snoring and contribute to sleep apnea. Nasal conditions known to cause snoring include nasal valve collapse, septal deviation, enlarged turbinates, nasal polyps, sinusitis, and nasal tumor. There are specific surgical procedures to correct each of these problems. Most of these procedures can be done in a doctor's office or in an outpatient surgical center. Patients who have nasal surgery can resume work immediately, or certainly within two or three days following the procedure. Although pain after the surgery is minimal, there may be some temporary discomfort, dripping, or stuffiness.

Nasal Valve Collapse

Nasal valve collapse refers to collapse of the cartilage supporting the tip of the nose. When you breathe in, and the cartilage is too weak to hold up against the airflow, it collapses. This is seen frequently in an older person's nose or in those who have had cosmetic surgery on the nose (rhinoplasty).

Nasal valve collapse can be corrected by using external nasal strips that hold the nose open (as mentioned in Chapter 7) or surgically adding cartilage to the nasal tip. This surgical procedure is called *nasal reconstruction* and is performed in the operating room under general or local anesthesia. Cartilage is taken from the nasal septum or ear and used to support the nasal tip. This prevents further collapse and improves the nasal airway.

Deviated Septum

The nasal septum is the wall that divides the inside of the nose into two halves. A *deviated septum* occurs when the cartilage and bone of the nasal septum have bent into the airway, causing obstruction and increased resistance to airflow. A deviated septum may be hereditary or caused by trauma. A severe deviation of the septum may cause you to snore or have disturbed sleep.

Surgery to correct the deviation structurally opens and widens the nasal airway and is performed in an operating room under general anesthesia or local anesthesia with sedation. The surgery removes or straightens the bent cartilage. There is no change to the outside appearance of your nose, and you will have no external bruising or swelling. You may go home the same day and experience very little pain or discomfort.

Turbinate Hypertrophy

Enlargement of the turbinates, resulting from swelling of their mucous membranes, can also cause nasal obstruction. Whether caused by allergy, irritation, or infection, the enlarged turbinates make it difficult to breathe and increase snoring. That is why snoring is a common occurence when you have a cold. Continued irritation of the turbinates, known as *rhinitis*, causes prolonged enlargement (*turbinate hypertrophy*) and leads to nasal obstruction and snoring.

Turbinate hypertrophy is treated surgically by decreasing the size of the turbinates using electric cautery (an electric device that cuts tissue and burns blood vessels) or a laser. The doctor may remove all or part of the turbinate. This procedure is done in the operating room under local or general anesthesia and is often combined with correction of the septum.

Nasal Polyps

Nasal polyps are grape-like swellings of the nasal tissue associated with allergy and irritation. In most cases, polyps are benign (noncancerous) tissue but should be removed because they cause nasal obstruction and block the sinuses, predisposing them to infection.

Polyps are removed in the operating room under general anesthesia or local anesthesia with sedation. The procedure is done through the nose using the same technique as sinus surgery.

Chronic Sinusitis

Sinuses are air spaces in the skull bone around the eyes and nose that are lined by a mucous membrane. The sinuses communicate with the nose and throat through ducts. Inflammation of this membrane due to infection or allergy causes sinusitis. *Chronic sinusitis* that does not respond to medical management may cause snoring because the nasal airway is obstructed by the swollen tissues. You might have facial pain, dental pain, discolored nasal secretions, and bad breath from sinusitis.

The diagnosis is made by examination, and sometimes a computerized tomography scan is ordered when the doctor thinks surgery should be considered. The surgery is done in the operating room under general anesthesia or local anesthesia with sedation. Using a telescope, the surgeon will look inside the nose and then remove the infected tissue and polyps, restoring the normal drainage pathway of the sinuses. The telescope allows the surgeon an excellent view of the sinuses. Infected or abnormal tissue structures can be removed with special forceps or by laser. The procedure is not painful and does not cause external bruising or swelling, and you may go home the same day or the next day. For the best results, careful follow-up is required for the next few weeks, but you can probably go back to work within three or four days.

Nasal Tumors

Nasal tumors are rare but can cause nasal obstruction. Tumors may be benign (noncancerous) or malignant (cancerous) and are diagnosed by a complete nasal examination. Removal of the tumor removes the obstruction and cures snoring.

It should be noted that after tumor removal it may be necessary to repair the nose or improve the air passages inside the nose to help you adapt to using nasal CPAP.

TONSILLECTOMY AND ADENOIDECTOMY

The tonsils and adenoids are made of lymphoid tissue and are part of the immune system. The tonsils are located on the side of the throat, while the adenoids are located behind the nose and above the soft palate. The tonsils and adenoids act as filters guarding the entrance to the lower respiratory system. They remove viruses, bacteria, and particles in inspired air. Sometimes they become clogged, swollen, and infected. In the 1960s, adenoid and tonsil enlargement was recognized as a cause of sleep apnea and snoring. Since that time, many reports have documented very large tonsils and adenoids as the cause of airway obstruction and snoring in adults and children.

Adenoid enlargement causing nasal obstruction is the most common cause of snoring in children. Extreme enlargement of the tonsils can cause snoring and sleep apnea, and is the most common cause of sleep apnea in children. The tonsils, adenoids, or both are removed if they are chronically infected or contribute to sleep apnea. Removal usually stops the snoring and decreases the apnea. However, the tonsils and adenoids are usually not removed for snoring alone. Rarely, a tumor of the tonsils or adenoids is the cause of snoring. The doctor will diagnose this during a physical examination, and removal of the tumor usually cures the snoring.

Tonsillectomy and *adenoidectomy* are usually performed in the operating room under general anesthesia. Both the tonsils and adenoids are removed through the mouth. The tonsils are removed by cutting the tissue away from the underlying muscle, using an electric cautery, laser, snare, or knife. All methods give similar results. Adenoids are removed by a specially designed instrument that passes through the mouth into the nose. Both procedures carry a risk of bleeding.

UVULOPALATOPHARYNGOPLASTY

If the site of airway obstruction is the palate, uvula, and tonsils (the oropharynx), the doctor will consider surgery. The uvulopalatopharyngoplasty (UPPP) (tailoring or trimming of the size of the back of the throat) was described in 1952 by a Japanese doctor as a treatment for sleep apnea. It was brought to the United States in 1981 and since then has been modified by numerous doctors.

UPPP continues to be the most commonly performed procedure for sleep apnea and is effective at reducing obstructive sleep apnea and eliminating snoring.

The effectiveness of UPPP has been demonstrated repeatedly in the majority of carefully selected people whose level of airway obstruction is in the oropharynx. For those with moderate to severe sleep apnea, this procedure has success rates ranging from 33 to 63 percent for sleep apnea and over 80 percent for snoring. In one series of studies, UPPP resulted in a greater than 50 percent reduction in the apnea/hypopnea index in 70 percent of the people. Reduction or elimination of snoring was reported by up to 87 percent of patients. Keep in mind that UPPP is used primarily for sleep apnea and is usually not the surgical choice for snoring without sleep apnea.

UPPP is done in the hospital operating room under general anesthesia. The procedure involves removing most of the soft palate, uvula, and tonsils using an electrocautery, laser, or knife (see Figure 8.1). The result is a wider oral airway and reduced obstruction. Count on spending one to two days in the hospital so that you can be provided with fluids and pain medications and monitored for breathing difficulty.

Although UPPP is a valuable procedure, occasionally there may be significant complications. Pain is the most common problem and may be quite severe. Pain may decrease the desire to drink fluids, which can lead to dehydration. Hospitalization for administration of intravenous fluids and pain medication may be required, and bleeding may occur. In some people, a change in speech may occur. In particular, loss of the ability to make sounds such as a "rolling r" may be a problem, especially for language teachers and singers. Nasal regurgitation of liquids (usually temporary) may occur. Airway loss, throat swelling, and death are rare but have occurred.

The possible complications associated with this procedure, and the resultant hospitalization and specialized monitoring, have limited its use to the more serious condition of sleep apnea. UPPP is now considered overtreatment for snoring without sleep apnea. Patients who undergo this type of surgery *must* have repeat poly-

FIGURE 8.1

UVULOPALATOPHARYNGOPLASTY (UPPP)

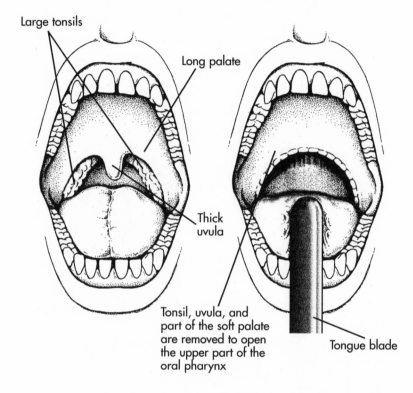

Large tonsils

Long palate

Thick uvula

Tonsil, uvula, and part of the soft palate are removed to open the upper part of the oral pharynx

Tongue blade

somnography after the operation to be certain that their sleep-related breathing disorder is better and not worse. Some may be converted from snoring apneic patients into nonsnoring apneic patients who no longer have the warning sign of snoring.

LASER-ASSISTED UVULOPALATOPLASTY

Laser-assisted uvulopalatoplasty (LAUP) is a new and effective method for treating habitual snoring. It was invented by a French physician, Dr. Yves-Victor Kamani, in 1988 and was brought to the

FIGURE 8.2

LASER-ASSISTED UVULOPALATOPLASTY (LAUP)

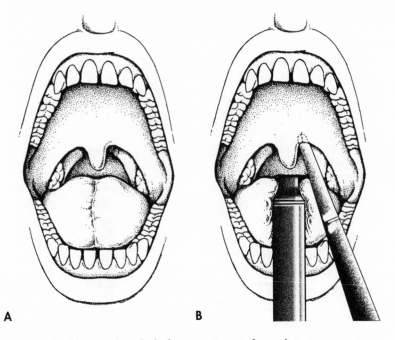

A   **B**

A. The soft palate and uvula before LAUP is performed. **B.** Laser cutting the soft palate to remove the floppy tissue.

United States in 1991. Since that time, it has been modified by U.S. physicians and is now a commonly performed procedure.

LAUP is reserved for those who have simple or pure snoring and mild sleep apnea. The procedure is performed under local anesthesia in a physician's office using a carbon dioxide (CO_2) laser. The laser is used to enlarge the oral airway by reshaping the uvula and palate (see Figure 8.2). LAUP may be used for moderate sleep apnea but only in a hospital setting or monitored surgery center.

When snoring and airway obstruction are determined to be caused by the palate and uvula, LAUP is the best surgical procedure. A person with a long uvula and excessive palatal tissue causing the

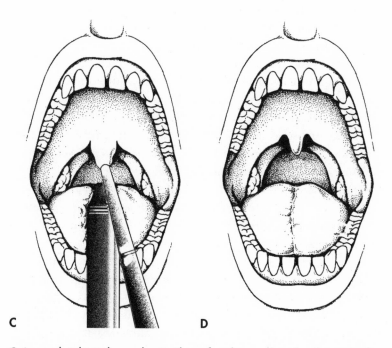

C. Laser shrinking the uvula. **D.** The soft palate and uvula after LAUP has been performed.

snoring is definitely a candidate for this type of surgery. Because other sites of obstruction do *not* respond to LAUP, a complete evaluation is needed to determine the appropriateness of the procedure.

LAUP is a series of procedures removing small amounts of the palate and uvula to shorten, stiffen, and reshape the tissue. The CO_2 laser is used to vaporize the structures during each procedure. Usually three to five visits are required to achieve the result. With multiple procedures spaced at intervals of four to six weeks, the risk of complications from removing too much palate is avoided, and the discomfort, if any, is minimal.

LAUP is done right in the doctor's office. You will sit upright in a chair, and the mouth will be anesthetized with an oral spray and then an injection. The laser is then used to shorten the uvula and vaporize the palate on each side of the uvula. This takes between ten and thirty minutes, and you may return to normal activities after the procedure. You may experience some soreness or discomfort in the throat for up to ten days, which occasionally is severe. This is usually relieved with oral pain medications. The doctor will tell you not to ingest alcohol, spicy foods, and citrus juice, to avoid irritating the palate.

The second procedure is performed after the palate has healed, usually four to six weeks after the first procedure. Each subsequent procedure is performed in a similar fashion to the first.

Complications of LAUP are rare but may occur. Bleeding occurs in about 2 percent of patients and is usually controlled by cauterization in the office. Infection, narrowing of the nasal passage, and voice change are rare but have occurred.

LAUP has been shown to be *85 percent* effective in eliminating snoring or reducing it to a more tolerable level. Some people with mild sleep apnea may benefit from LAUP by an improvement in the quality of sleep. One major advantage of LAUP over UPPP (see Table 8.2) is the ability to remove tissue gradually without the risk of cutting away too much. LAUP may also be combined with other procedures, depending on the cause of obstruction and snoring.

RADIOFREQUENCY TISSUE VOLUME REDUCTION

Using a special instrument, the surgeon can deliver radiofrequency energy to tissues such as the palate, uvula, and tongue. This energy generates low heat that gently burns the tissue underneath the skin or mucous membrane. This results in shrinkage of the structures and enlargement of the airway. The surgeon can regulate the heat disbursement from the radiofrequency signal to control the amount of tissue that will ultimately shrink.

Radiofrequency procedures are effective and safe. This type of

| TABLE 8.2 | | | |

Uvulopalatopharyngoplasty (UPPP) versus Laser-Assisted Uvulopalatoplasty (LAUP)

INDICATIONS	PROCEDURE REQUIREMENTS	NO. OF PROCED- URES	POTENTIAL COMPLI- CATIONS
UPPP			
Used for moderate to severe sleep apnea	Hospital, 1–2 days General anesthesia	1	Airway com- promise Pain, bleeding Change in speech Problems swallowing
LAUP			
Used for snoring and mild sleep apnea	Office, outpatient Local anesthesia	3–5	Mild pain Minor bleeding

tissue volume reduction can be done under local anesthesia on an outpatient basis at specialized medical centers. You may need repeated treatments as for LAUP until the optimal results are achieved. As with the other types of surgery, it is important that the doctor evaluate your situation to make sure you are a good candidate for radiofrequency procedures.

MAXILLOFACIAL SURGERY

In a number of people, the tongue is the anatomical cause of airway obstruction, snoring, and sleep apnea. If this is your problem, the doctor can use one of several methods to reduce the size of the tongue or to advance the jaw and create more room for the tongue. It should be noted that there are only a few surgeons around the country who have the very special expertise in doing these operations. These methods include the following:

Uvulopalatopharyngoglossoplasty—an operation that incorporates a modified UPPP with limited removal of tissue.

Midline glossectomy and linguoplasty—two procedures that create an enlargement in the airway at the back of the tongue. In midline glossectomy, a laser is used to cut out a 2.5-centimeter by 5.0-centemeter rectangular strip from the back half of the tongue. In some cases, surrounding tissue in the hypopharynx is reduced in size by the laser.

Linguoplasty—a procedure different from midline glossectomy in that additional tissue is cut away further back and to the side of the portion excised in midline glossectomy.

The main side effects of these operations on the tongue include bleeding, which requires some extra treatment, and pain or difficulty swallowing, which lasts two to three weeks.

Other more complicated surgical procedures may be helpful to increase the size of the airway space behind the tongue. These include genioglossus advancement with hyoid myotomy (GAHM) and maxillomandibular advancement osteotomy (MMO). Both procedures are usually done at very specialized medical centers as a last resort to cure snoring and sleep apnea. The doctor can explain each in detail.

TRACHEOSTOMY

Tracheostomy was the first surgical treatment for sleep apnea. It is used to surgically bypass all sites of airway obstruction. Currently, it is used only in extremely obese patients who cannot tolerate nasal CPAP, for reasons described on pages 98–100. It is often recommended for life-threatening sleep apnea that does not respond to conservative management.

If the doctor recommends this type of surgery, you and your family will be counseled on tracheostomy care and the psychosocial implications. The surgery is performed in the operating room under general anesthesia. An incision is made in the middle of the neck to expose the trachea (breathing tube). A small opening is made in the trachea, and a tracheostomy tube is inserted. You breathe through the open tube in the neck while you sleep but plug the tube during the day so you can speak. The tube is small enough to allow air to enter the trachea from above into the pharynx and larynx and down into the lungs.

After the procedure, you will be monitored in the hospital until the airway is secure, usually for three to four days. Both you and your family are taught to clean and suction the tube at home. The tracheostomy tube can be removed when it is no longer needed, such as after weight loss or if and when you decide to use nasal CPAP.

EACH PERSON IS DIFFERENT

It's important to remember that each person is different. While this book cannot replace a proper and accurate medical diagnosis, it does explain the many ways snoring can be stopped. In the next chapter, we introduce you to several people who snored and explain how they were able to cure their snoring and get a good night's sleep once more.

CHAPTER 9

Silent Nights

re you *sure* this really works?" That's a common question. While you finally understand why stopping snoring is vital for good health and longevity, perhaps you also wonder if the snoring cure will work in your situation.

Every day at the Cleveland Clinic we see people who are taking measures to cure snoring and subsequently, enjoy a better quality of life. For example, after forty-six-year-old Richard was diagnosed with obstructive sleep apnea and successfully started continuous positive airway pressure using nasal CPAP at night, he reported feeling younger, having more energy, and even being more productive at home and work. "My wife even thinks I'm fun to be around!" Richard shared.

Carolyn, a fifty-four-year-old registered nurse, also used the four-step cure after she was diagnosed with pure snoring. Losing twenty pounds along with reducing nasal congestion with a steroid nasal spray helped her to stop snoring and feel more energetic and alert.

After using the four steps described in this book, thousands of our patients now attest to increased energy and daytime productivity, as well as improved mood and outlook on life. Yet if you snore or have obstructive sleep apnea, it might be difficult to see the hope of an actual cure. Sometimes you might feel as if you are the "only one" who tosses and turns all night and feels sleepy the next day. Knowing that other people have experienced the annoy-ing and sometimes dangerous symptoms, yet have succeeded in "curing" these can be most encouraging.

Let the following four stories of "Silent Nights" give you addi-tional impetus to get control of your nighttime noise and *stop snor-ing once and for all!*

A BEDTIME STORY WITH A HAPPY ENDING

Charles is a fifty-three-year-old man who had a good job, many friends, and a wife who adored him. However, over the last few months, he complained of being "too tired to enjoy life." Charles thought that his fatigue was attributable to stress because it wors-ened after the firm he worked for was sold to a large corporation with headquarters in another state. After catching himself dozing at work one day, Charles began to worry that he might become a victim of downsizing. He went to his local doctor who suggested that he exercise more and lose some weight to boost his daytime energy and alertness.

Realizing his great distress, Charles's wife insisted that he also see a specialist at the Cleveland Clinic. During the initial examina-tion Charles was asked about the length and quality of his sleep, and it turned out that even if he slept for longer hours on the weekend, he still was exhausted. His wife accompanied him to the interview and said that Charles snored and grunted loudly when he dozed off in his lounge chair while trying to watch the early evening news. She had always taken his snoring for granted, because she usually fell asleep before he did and was not awakened by the nighttime noise.

Further questioning revealed that Charles frequently awoke in the morning with a dry mouth and a headache. The specialist sus-pected that the quality of the sleep Charles was getting was very poor. It was fragmented by repeated episodes of obstruction in the upper airway called *apneas*, which were ended by brief arousals. The arousals were not long enough to awaken him completely from his slumber, but they did fragment or ruin his sleep, leaving him essentially sleep deprived.

At the Cleveland Clinic's sleep disorder laboratory, Charles had a sleep study called a *polysomnography* (see page 141). These tests confirmed the suspicion that he had obstructive sleep apnea. He was not getting the deep, uninterrupted sleep that he needed to feel rested.

Different treatment options were discussed but because his sleep apnea was fairly severe, it was decided that nasal CPAP (see page 94) was the best treatment for him. Charles was shown how the nasal CPAP machine worked, and he tried on a mask during the day at the clinic. Using the nasal CPAP, he was able to breathe fairly comfortably, so he was scheduled for another sleep study in the laboratory. During the second sleep study, Charles slept with the nasal CPAP, and the exact pressure required to prevent the apneas was determined.

Later that week, the machine, mask, and accessories were delivered to his home. After sleeping while using the nasal CPAP machine for just a few nights, Charles's family and friends noticed a big difference in his mood. Not only did he feel more energetic and alert during the day, he was able to exercise and ride his bicycle around the subdivision where he lived. Charles's life, like his personality, returned to normal. He was sleeping soundly with the nasal CPAP and awakened refreshed each morning. For someone with sleep apnea, this was a very happy ending for the story!

THE SNORE HEARD ROUND THE WORLD

Sandra, age forty-seven, worked as the social director on a cruise ship that frequently made long voyages around the world. Sandra was well liked by everyone on the ship, felt quite well, and was an excellent employee. Yet to her dismay, the crew members who slept near her cabin complained about her loud and very obnoxious snoring.

On one trip, the cabin above Sandra's was occupied by a retired otolaryngologist (ENT specialist) and his wife. One morning at about 5:30, she was awakened by a gentle knock on the door. Imagine Sandra's embarrassment when it was the doctor's wife. This woman expressed great concern about the snoring that she had been hearing when she walked by Sandra's cabin on the way to her early-morning yoga class. Since the doctor's wife had proofread a number of articles her husband had written, she knew the potential significance of snoring and recommended that Sandra go for a consultation when she was in a major port city.

Luckily for Sandra, she took this advice. She wound up undergoing a sleep study that revealed very mild sleep apnea and mainly loud snoring. The sleep medicine doctor recommended that she consider laser-assisted uvulopalatoplasty (LAUP), and Sandra went to a surgeon who was experienced in doing this operation.

After several laser treatment sessions in his office, Sandra borrowed a special tape recorder to record the sounds of her breathing during her next brief cruise. When she returned the tape to the doctor, she was delighted to report that the crew on the ship said they had not had such quiet nights in a very long time. The tape recording confirmed their statements.

THE MYSTERIOUS HEADACHE

More than a month after being hit in the head with a racquetball racquet, Harvey, a forty-seven-year-old software designer, was still having severe headaches. The headaches seemed to be getting worse and were occurring more frequently, making it difficult for him to concentrate on his work. He was also experiencing ongoing fatigue, even when he slept for hours on the weekend. In the past few weeks, Harvey said he was drinking more and more coffee in the morning "just to barely function," and in the afternoon, he kept a large glass of strong iced tea or caffeinated cola at his workstation so that he would not doze.

A couple of months prior to his head injury, Harvey had experienced a spell of severe sleepiness. When he dozed off and knocked a glass of tea over on his computer keyboard, both he and his wife became concerned about his health. Yet a complete medical examination, including a computerized tomography scan of his brain, failed to show anything abnormal. The severe headaches sent him back to the doctor but another work-up still did not reveal a cause for the headaches and fatigue.

Harvey was starting to feel that "it was all in his head," and this bothered him even more than the pain and the fatigue. He knew the symptoms were not figments of his imagination and had difficulty accepting that nothing was wrong with him. He became depressed and angry and finally his doctor sent him for another opinion.

At the Cleveland Clinic, Harvey was seen by a psychologist. He had such difficulty concentrating that he could not get through the battery of tests he was asked to take, especially those designed to assess his memory. When Harvey began to doze off during a simple questionnaire inquiring about his sex life, the psychologist referred him to one of the sleep disorder specialists.

During the initial interview, the specialist found out that Harvey's wife had congenital deafness, so she could not report on whether or not he snored. Because of his headaches and daytime sleepiness, he underwent an overnight sleep study, which revealed that he had many episodes of obstructive sleep apneas and hypopneas at a rate of almost one per minute of sleep. Most of the obstructive events occurred when he was sleeping on his back.

During this period of testing, the psychologist was arranging for Harvey to start taking some antidepressant medications but kept Harvey off the medicines while he tried positional therapy designed to help him avoid sleeping on his back. After two weeks, Harvey felt more rested in the morning and was drinking less cof-

fee and tea throughout the course of the day. His mood was better, and he even decided to get back on the racquetball court with
a protective helmet. Harvey and his wife went for a brief vacation,
and upon returning, he completed a complicated software program
he had been struggling with for a long time. The headaches never
returned.

A NEW FOCUS ON HEALTH . . .
NOT ON WEIGHT

Cathy, a twenty-eight-year-old newlywed, was in relatively good
health except that at five feet, three inches tall, she tipped the scales
at 170 pounds. She went to a dietitian to discuss her weight problem, and during the interview, she revealed that her husband complained about her loud snoring. Instead of exercising each day, she
admitted that lately, she spent a good part of the time sitting on a
bench at the park watching her husband and the other runners
whiz by. This young woman conveyed to the dietitian that she was
becoming increasingly unhappy about her weight, lack of energy,
and snoring. She helped pay the bills and was contributing to their
savings for a house in an upscale neighborhood closer to the down-
town area where they worked. However, her stressful job did not
pay well and required long and irregular hours. Her meals often
included "fast or junk foods," which she grabbed at the cafeteria or
from a street vendor. She felt out of control of her situation.

The dietitian suggested she attend one-hour weekly group
counseling sessions. During the first few sessions, the patients
focused on what health meant to them and how they could
achieve their maximal health potential. They soon realized that if
they were to be successful, they needed to change their eating
habits. They were advised to keep a food diary to review at a subsequent session. It became quite clear that most of them were
underestimating the amount of food that they were consuming.
Then, they were advised to control the amount of high-calorie
foods that they were eating by keeping the number of daily calo-

ries no more than ten times their desired body weight. For another session they were told to try to estimate the amount of exercise they thought they were getting on a daily basis. While keeping a diary it also became apparent that they had a tendency to *overestimate* the amount of exercise that they were actually doing. Each participant in the group decided on an exercise program that seemed best for him or her and on a daily calorie goal. The dietitian encouraged them to lose weight slowly, at a rate of one or at most two pounds each week.

Cathy was enthusiastic about this sensible plan to losing weight and began to set her goals. She started her jogging routine even though at first she could not go as fast as she had previously because she was out of shape and heavier. She also bought an insulated lunch bag and began to pack healthy, calorie-conscious lunches for herself. Within a few months, Cathy found that her weight was approaching a more desirable level and that she could jog better than she could in quite some time. Her husband, who worked in a building a few blocks away, started to call her shortly before each lunch hour to request that they meet for a brief picnic lunch at a park nearby. Soon, he also was packing his own health-conscious lunch.

Along with wearing clothes several sizes smaller, Cathy told of another great benefit: Her husband did not complain any more about her snoring. She seemed to have a lot more energy during the day and was able to take on a different position at work that was less stressful.

By focusing on her health and desire to be fit rather than on food, Cathy was able to lose weight and adopt a healthier lifestyle that was personally more rewarding.

....

CHAPTER 10

Questions You Might Ask

E ffective communication with your doctor could save your life, especially if your snoring is associated with uncontrolled blood pressure or sleep apnea. At the Cleveland Clinic, it is our experience that many people wait too long before seeking an accurate diagnosis for their snoring. After you read this book, we encourage you to write down questions you may have regarding snoring, including specific risk factors and modes of treatment, then talk with your doctor about these concerns. Once you understand how snoring affects your health, you can take immediate measures to stop it altogether.

The following represent answers to questions we hear most frequently from those who are actively seeking a cure for snoring:

Q. When is referral to a sleep specialist indicated?

A. If you have loud snoring, witnessed breath-holding spells, and daytime fatigue or sleepiness, then talk to your doctor about a referral to a sleep specialist. You would be a good candidate for confirmatory polysomnography, as described in Chapter 5. Most of the cost of this sleep study is covered by insurance.

Q. My husband is a mouth breather and is always congested in the morning. How does this affect his continual snoring?

A. Your husband's mouth breathing is due to nasal congestion caused by allergy or infection. This may result in a *dry* mouth in the morning. When he breathes in through his mouth, the rate at which air enters the trachea is reduced, because there is more resistance to air entering the back of his throat from the mouth than from his nose. Also, enlarged tonsils or an excessively long soft palate may contribute to narrowing at the back of the throat, adding to the resistance. This increased resistance creates problems as the air pressure at the back of the throat has to be even lower in relationship to atmospheric pressure in order for air to get in. As a result, the respiratory muscles, mainly the *diaphragm*, have to work harder and harder to generate the lower pressures. Also, the muscles in the upper airway, such as those that keep the tongue from blocking the back of the throat and those that keep the lower throat open at the entrance to the trachea, have to be more active to maintain an open airway. During sleep these muscles relax and the throat narrows, causing snoring and worsening apnea. Even though one may take pride in being fit and flexible, sometimes there may be a lack of coordination between the breathing muscles and the muscles that maintain the opening at the entrance to the main airway.

Q. What are the health risks of untreated obstructive sleep apnea?

A. Obstructive sleep apnea carries a significant risk of medical complications, including high blood pressure, myocardial infarction (heart attack), abnormal heart rhythms, congestive heart failure, and stroke. In addition, the potential for crippling or fatal motor-vehicle or industrial accidents is much higher because of the excessive daytime sleepiness. Read Chapter 3 for more information on obstructive sleep apnea, then talk with your doctor about the suggested cures such as weight loss (see Chapter 6) and nasal continuous positive airway pressure (CPAP) (see Chapter 7).

Q. What are the common treatment alternatives for obstructive sleep apnea?

A. A person with mild obstructive sleep apnea may respond well to using an oral appliance (see page 93) or to weight loss. Moderate to severe obstructive sleep apneas are best treated with nasal CPAP (see page 94) or upper-airway surgery (see Chapter 8).

Q. Who might be a candidate for weight-reduction surgical treatment?

A. In 1991, the National Institutes of Health outlined the indications for surgical treatment based on a study by a panel of experts. These experts stated that someone who has a body mass index (BMI) greater than 40 (see page 58) or a BMI greater than 35 in combination with life-threatening problems such as severe diabetes mellitus, high blood pressure, obstructive sleep apnea, or coronary artery disease *may* be a candidate for this kind of aggressive treatment for obesity.

If you are overweight, reread Chapter 6 and see if the practical methods of increasing exercise and calorie control can help your situation. If your BMI is in the dangerous range (see pages 60–61), talk to your doctor about a monitored weight-loss plan. It may be helpful to talk with a certified nutritionist about dietary modifications.

Q. I have been told that I have horrendous snoring but I seem to sleep just fine, and I feel well during the day. Nonetheless, my wife won't stay in the same bed with me. What can I do about it?

A. The most important thing to do first is to make sure that the snoring is *not* a symptom of obstructive sleep apnea. This usually requires a consultation with a physician specially trained and experienced in the diagnosis and treatment of sleep disorders. A sleep study called *polysomnography* (see page 141) will be done to monitor your breathing pattern, oxygen levels, and sleep quality. If it turns out that you have *pure* snoring without any sleep apnea or that you have *extremely mild* obstructive sleep apnea, then you should be examined by an otolaryngologist (ENT specialist) experienced in surgery of the upper airway for snoring. Nowadays, you are most likely to be offered a laser-assisted uvulopalatoplasty (see page 109) for relief of your loud snoring. Patients with pure snoring (no sleep apnea at all) or very mild obstructive sleep apnea are good candidates for laser-assisted uvulopalatoplasty. There are cures for snoring, so using this book as a guide, do not stop until you've found the right solution for your situation.

Q. My nine-year-old son sleeps in a peculiar position, with his head and neck extended far backward most of the time. When he does not sleep like this, he has very loud snoring. Do I need to worry about this and what can be done about his snoring?

A. Most normal children snore at one time or another and many, particularly those with nasal allergies, snore almost every night. Snoring that is regular—without interruptions by breath holding, labored breathing, or the taking of unusual postures during sleep, or with a lot of sweating—is not likely to represent a serious problem. However, if any of these signs are present along with a slow growth rate, bed-wetting, daytime sleepiness, or problems in school, then further evaluation is necessary. Your son should be seen by a pediatrician well versed in sleep disorders of children.

Q. Our twelve-year-old daughter is small for her age, snores loudly, and recently started to wet her bed. Do you think there is a problem we need to bring to our doctor's attention?

A. In contrast to the adult population with obstructive sleep apnea, the majority of children with sleep apnea are often underweight and may fail to grow at a normal rate. This retarded growth may be a result of poor appetite, difficulty swallowing, increased work of breathing, or insufficient growth hormone. Growth hormone is secreted at relatively high levels during the deepest stages of sleep (stages 3 and 4). These stages may be reduced or absent in patients with significant sleep apnea (see page 8), including children. Bed-wetting may be a symptom of obstructive sleep apnea in a child.

Talk to your pediatrician about your concerns and see if a sleep disorder specialist can evaluate your daughter. There are many methods of treating this in children, so seek answers until you feel her sleep is normal.

Q. What is the most common cause of obstructive sleep apnea in children?

A. Enlargement of the tonsils, the adenoids, or both is the most common cause of obstructive sleep apnea in children. Removal of these organs relieves the obstruction in most children with the problem.

Q. How can I find a physician who is truly expert in the field of sleep disorders so I can get the best possible cure for my snoring?

A. Doctors who have had special training in the field of sleep disorders and who have passed a qualifying examination are certified by the American Board of Sleep Medicine. A directory of these doctors can be obtained from the American Sleep Disorders Association in Rochester, Minnesota. (See Resources.)

Q. Are there any good medicines that can help me lose weight?

A. A variety of drugs related to amphetamines help decrease appetite or increase energy usage, but these may be associated with dangerous side effects, particularly in people who have cardiovascular disease. Other medications that are related to antidepressant medications do not raise blood pressure or the rate at which food is metabolized. Some of these drugs cause pulmonary hypertension and valvular heart disease. Moreover, whenever patients stop taking these drugs, they regain weight promptly. A lot of research is ongoing, as scientists continue to look for the ideal, safe medicine for the control of weight. But in the meantime, be skeptical of quick fixes for obesity. Modifications in diet, exercise, and lifestyle, though very challenging to implement and maintain, must always be a main part of prevention and treatment.

Q. How much weight do I need to lose before I will see an improvement in my snoring and sleep apnea?

A. A loss of 10 to 20 percent of your weight, if you are significantly overweight, will result in an improvement and possible cure of your snoring and sleep apnea.

Q. I stopped snoring last year but am having difficult staying asleep through the night. Are there some tips you can offer on how to get quality sleep?

A. If you have no physiological problem, then you might try the following suggestions to guarantee a more restful sleep:

1. Sleep only as much as needed to feel refreshed and healthy the following day. (Curtailing the time you spend in bed seems to solidify sleep; excessively long times in bed seem related to fragmented and shallow sleep.)

2. Eat less sugar, which can cause sudden increases and dips in blood sugar levels. (When your blood sugar level drops, it may cause you to awaken in the middle of the night.)

3. Avoid stimulants such as caffeine and nicotine.

4. A steady daily amount of exercise seems to deepen sleep, but do not exercise right before bedtime as it may increase alertness.

5. Make sure your bedroom is soundproofed, or wear ear plugs, if you are bothered by noises while sleeping. (Some people find help with "white noise"—a humming sound produced by a machine or the static from a radio when a station has gone off the air.)

6. Eat foods that are high in carbohydrates, such as breads, cereal, pasta, or sherbet, to raise the level of serotonin in the brain. (Serotonin is a mood-elevating chemical in the body that produces a calming effect.)

7. Avoid alcohol before bedtime. (Even though it relaxes you, the sleep will be fragmented or of poor quality.)

8. Take a hot bath about three hours before bedtime, then keep the temperature in your bedroom cool. (Sleep usually follows the cooling phase of your body's temperature cycle.)

9. Spend time outdoors each day, especially during the morning hours, to keep your body's circadian rhythms in harmony.

10. Have peace of mind, using prayer or meditation to let your worries go each night.

Q. If I want to reach a certain weight, how many calories may I eat each day?

A. In order to reach a "target weight" you must control your intake. If your desired weight is, for example, 130 pounds, then you are supposed to eat only 1,300 calories each day. In other words, you should only consume ten times (in calories) your target weight (in pounds).

Q. How much exercise should I try to get each day?

A. You should exercise as much as you are comfortable doing after consulting with your doctor. It is generally recommended, however, that you *accumulate* at least thirty minutes of moderately intense physical activity every day of the week. This is the equivalent of a brisk twenty-minute walk and ten minutes of walking up stairs or swimming laps. If you do this, then you will burn an extra 200 or so calories per day and over the course of a year you could lose twenty pounds.

Q. If I have obstructive sleep apnea, may I drive a car?

A. The laws regulating this vary according to the state in which you live. However, common sense and ethical considerations (concern for the well-being of yourself and those around you) would suggest that you not operate a motor vehicle or other dangerous machinery until your daytime sleepiness is improved.

Q. I am having trouble adjusting to my nasal CPAP mask and I tend to pull it off in the middle of the night, or I just cannot fall asleep with it. What can I do?

A. Make an appointment with the sleep specialist who pre-scribed the nasal CPAP and bring all of your equipment with you so that proper fit and function can be verified. Then assuming that your nose is not in need of some treatment for congestion, a peri-od of acclimatization or desensitization must be started. This requires that you practice wearing the mask and breathing with the nasal CPAP when you are awake. This acclimatization is like break-ing in a new pair of shoes. Learning as much as you can about sleep apnea and its consequences if untreated will help you get more motivated to use the system. Also, trying variations of the mask and machine may be quite helpful.

Q. My doctor was trying to explain how air pressure changes actual-ly cause the obstruction in the airway, but the explanation was over my head. Can you help me to understand this?

A. How air flows through your upper airway will depend on several factors. These factors include the shape or dimensions of the airway itself and the function of the muscles surrounding it that help keep it open.

Did you know that air is pushed into your nose and mouth by the force of atmospheric pressure? This happens because the pres-sure inside the respiratory system during normal inspiration is below atmospheric pressure. From the tip of the nose to the upper airway, air is pushed down the conducting airways—the trachea and larger main bronchi—to the lungs, which are really only passive airbags. If there is increased resistance to airflow in the oropharynx because of anatomic narrowing, then the pressure in the upper air-way will drop and tend to get further below the atmospheric level. If at any point in the oropharynx the pressure inside is far enough below the atmospheric level and the supporting muscles are not working enough to keep the airway open, then the airway will be pressed closed by the surrounding atmospheric pressure outside the airway. (See Figure 2.1, page 24, and Figure 7.1, page 83.)

Think about it this way. Remember years ago when paper straws were popular? Well, pretend you are sucking on a paper straw held tightly in your mouth. Point this straw up to the ceiling while sucking. What happens? Of course, the straw will tend to collapse closed. This happens because the pressure inside the straw is below the atmospheric pressure. This same reaction or closing of the airway occurs during obstructive sleep apneic events.

Q. I suffer from allergies year-round. I'm now on an inhaled steroid spray to try to reduce inflammation, but how does this inflammation cause me to snore at night?

A. Nasal congestion, either seasonal or perennial, can aggravate snoring. This occurs because increased resistance to airflow through the nose will result in a pressure at the back of the throat that is further below the atmospheric level, causing more of a tendency for the upper-airway walls to collapse in spite of the efforts of the various pharyngeal muscles to brace the airway open. The battle between pressure trying to close the airway and the muscles trying to prop it open will contribute to the fluttering of the structures and noise production. Different factors such as allergic or infectious rhinitis, sinusitis, a cold, or injury can cause nasal obstruction. If you are a mouth breather because of nasal congestion, then the chances that you snore are even greater. (Treatment for nasal congestion is discussed in Chapter 7.)

Q. While I have periodic snoring during a cold, I am bothered more by heartburn and awaken during the night with a burning feeling in my throat. Sometimes I have coughing spasms during sleep. Is this all related to a sleep disorder?

A. Heartburn or acid indigestion resulting from gastro-esophageal reflux is related to a sleep disorder. At times the efforts of the diaphragm pushing down on the abdominal contents, especially the stomach, are very great. This may cause increased pressure inside the stomach, with a resultant backwash of stomach acid into the esophagus or as high as the back of the throat. This bitter, burning, sour, acid taste or irritation can cause you to awaken abruptly out of a deep sleep. Sometimes, an asthma attack (spasm of the bronchial tubes in the lungs themselves with wheezing and shortness of breath) may be triggered.

Talk to your doctor about treatment for the heartburn or acid indigestion. There are prescription medications that work to reduce the acid in your stomach, allowing you to sleep soundly again.

Q. I have moderate obstructive sleep apnea according to a sleep study. During the examination, the doctor said I also have high blood pressure. Are these two problems related?

A. Systemic hypertension or high blood pressure is a common problem for more than 10 percent of the adult population. Not surprisingly, with the intricate connection between the heart and lungs, the correlation between systemic hypertension and sleep apnea is very strong. In fact, half of those with sleep apnea also have associated hypertension, while about a third of those who have hypertension can be shown after appropriate testing to also have sleep apnea.

This association between hypertension and sleep apnea is even stronger in people whose hypertension is difficult to control; half of those people will have sleep apnea. As the degree of sleep apnea worsens, the hypertension becomes more difficult to control. Once the underlying sleep apnea is recognized and treated, the hypertension can be more easily controlled by the usual medications.

The way sleep apnea leads to hypertension is thought to be by increased activity of certain hormones that are released in response to stress. Normally during sleep, especially the deeper stages, the blood pressure falls. During apneic events this normal decrease in blood pressure does not occur. If the apneas are severe, prolonged, and frequent, then the blood pressure may become elevated during sleep and then remain high during wakefulness.

When those with sleep apnea use nasal CPAP, the results are a consistent and sustained improvement in blood pressure control. Surprisingly, this positive benefit is seen after even a single night of therapy and is maintained as long as the person continues to use nasal CPAP. Many people with sleep apnea have realized successful control of their high blood pressure with less medicine or even without medications, once the sleep apnea was properly diagnosed and treated.

Q. How does high blood pressure associated with obstructive sleep apnea lead to heart disease?

A. The link between hypoxemia (low oxygen in the blood, which is caused by obstructive sleep apnea) and heart disease dates back to studies done in 1933 by Rothschild and Kissen. This information, along with the knowledge that people who have chronic lung disease are at increased risk of dying at night, has led to further studies that look at the consequences of nighttime *hypoxemia* on the cardiovascular system.

When normal people sleep, they have a 5 to 10 percent drop in both blood pressure and heart rate, compared to their awake state. (The *work of the heart and its oxygen and energy requirements* are determined by multiplying *your blood pressure by your heart rate*.) Therefore, when you are asleep, the work of your heart is normally decreased, and the heart is relatively protected from problems that otherwise might occur because of low oxygen levels.

If you have obstructive sleep apnea, you may try to take a breath but are unable to because of the upper-airway blockage. As a result, you try even harder to breathe in (as if trying to suck through a blocked straw), which produces negative pressure in the chest and around your heart. Blood in your vascular system returns to the heart more quickly as a result of this negative pressure in the chest. Many times, this load to the heart is increased because most people with obstructive sleep apnea have an increased blood volume resulting from obesity. The increase in the load of blood to the heart, along with the drop of oxygen content in the blood (which nourishes the heart) and the excess stress on the heart by the hypertensive response to the airway blockage, impacts negatively on cardiac function.

The rise in blood pressure during the apneic period (when breathing stops) and the drop in oxygen content in the blood worsen as the length of the apnea increases. Blood pressure may rise by 25 percent, and the oxygen content in the blood may drop as much as 5 to 25 percent during these periods.

Q. Can you have arrhythmias without having heart disease? Are arrhythmias or irregularities of heart rhythm a big concern for someone who has obstructive sleep apnea? How can these be avoided?

A. Arrhythmias or irregularities of the heart rhythm are frequent in sleeping individuals. Most commonly, bradycardia (a heart rate of less than sixty beats per minute) occurs. This is caused by a slowing of the electrical impulses in the heart that control its rate of pumping. Usually these types of arrhythmias are benign and do not have serious consequences. Nonetheless, when they occur too often or are more severe, they may be symptomatic and lead to complications. Symptoms include palpitations or chest discomfort, and complications can include problems such as fluid and salt retention, which in turn causes swelling or edema.

Treatment of obstructive sleep apnea either by nasal CPAP or even tracheostomy reduces the variability of the heart rate during apneic periods. Tracheostomy is a surgical procedure in which a tube is placed in a small opening in the trachea (Chapter 8). Resolution of the sleep apnea is associated with a reduction or ending of abnormal heart rates, rhythms, and extra beats. However, there is no definite proof that this translates into a decrease in sudden death.

Glossary

Acromegaly A disorder marked by a progressive enlargement of the head and face, hands and feet, and chest due to excessive amounts of growth hormone. It may be associated with OSA because of an abnormally formed upper airway.

Allergens Substances such as dust that trigger the body's allergic reaction and cause the nose to become runny or congested.

Alveoli Small sac-like structures located at the end of the bronchioles where the exchange of oxygen and carbon dioxide from the blood takes place.

Angina A severe, constricting pain in the chest due to a shortage of blood required to supply the heart muscle with oxygen.

Apnea The cessation of breathing that may occur during sleep.

Asthma A Greek word that Hippocrates used to describe episodes of shortness of breath. Today it refers to a disease marked by sudden, repeated attacks of shortness of breath due to narrowing of the bronchi. There may also be wheezing and cough.

BMI A common abbreviation for *body mass index*, which is calculated by dividing the body weight in kilograms by the height in meters squared, to get a measure of whether or not a person is overweight or has a risk factor for a disease such as OSA.

Bronchi   The airways that connect the windpipe (trachea) to the lungs.

Bronchioles   The smaller airways in the lungs.

Bruxism   A clenching or grinding of the teeth usually during sleep. Bruxism may be associated with OSA.

CPAP   A commonly used abbreviation for *continuous positive airway pressure*, which is used to relieve the obstruction in the oropharynx in patients with OSA.

CT   A commonly used abbreviation for *computerized tomography*, which is a special type of X ray imaging technique for getting detailed information about the anatomy in a particular part of the body such as the sinuses.

Diaphragm   The muscle that separates the chest cavity from the abdomen. It is the main provider of *inspiratory force* by expanding the size of the chest cavity. The diaphragm also lowers the pressure in the conducting airways in the lungs and up through the trachea to the oropharynx to below the atmospheric level so that air from the outside can be pushed in.

Hormone   A chemical substance formed in an organ or gland in the body that is secreted into the blood and carried to other organs or parts of the body. Hormones regulate the function and growth of various parts of the body.

Hypertension   A term used for *high blood pressure*. It usually is applied to the pressure in the arteries that carry blood from the left side of the heart to various parts of the body such as the brain, kidneys, digestive system, and muscles. This is called *systemic hypertension*. High blood pressure in the arteries that carry blood from the right side of the heart to the lungs is called *pulmonary hypertension*.

Hypothalamus A gland located at the base of the brain closely involved with the nervous system. The hypothalamus secretes hormones that regulate various body functions such as the release of other hormones from other glands in the body. It is involved in the control of appetite and body weight.

Hypothyroidism A condition in which the thyroid, a gland located under the skin in front of the neck, secretes abnormally low amounts of active hormone into the blood. This causes the body to use energy from food slower than normal, causing problems of weight gain or difficulty in losing weight.

Hypoxemia The technical term for low blood oxygen content, which may occur if air cannot get into the lungs because of a blockage in the upper airway as in an event of OSA. *Hypox* refers to "low levels of oxygen" and *emia* means "in the blood."

Insomnia A condition in which the person complains of difficulty falling asleep or problems staying asleep. Some people with OSA have a disorder of maintaining sleep caused by the severe arousals that end the apneas.

Larynx The organ of voice production located in the upper part of the respiratory system between the pharynx and the trachea. It includes the vocal cords.

Laser A device that produces a beam of high-energy light that can be used to shrink or burn tissue during a surgical procedure such as reduction of the size of the uvula and soft palate.

Lungs The main part of the respiratory system that takes oxygen from the air into the bloodstream and allows carbon dioxide to escape from the body.

Mandible The technical term for the jawbone.

Menopause The technical term for the permanent interruption of a woman's normal monthly menstrual periods.

MRI A commonly used abbreviation for *magnetic resonance imag-*

ing, which does not involve the use of radiation as in X rays but may be very useful in looking at a particular structure in the body.

Mucous membrane   A soft, pink, skin-like structure that lines many cavities and tubes in the body, such as the respiratory tract. The mucous membrane secretes a fluid containing mucus.

Mucus   A thick, slippery secretion produced by the mucous membrane that helps to lubricate and protect parts of the body such as the respiratory tract.

Nocturnal myoclonus   A repetitive jerking of an arm or more commonly one or both legs during sleep. It is also called *periodic limb movements of sleep* and may be associated with arousals that ruin sleep. It is particularly common after the age of forty. *Nocturnal* refers to "nighttime," *myo* means "muscle," and *clonus* is the technical term for "twitching."

Obesity   A condition in which a person is more than 20 percent overweight.

Oropharynx   The area extending from the level of the palate to the entrance of the larynx at the vocal cords. It is the collapsible region responsible for snoring and OSA.

OSA   A commonly used abbreviation for *obstructive sleep apnea.*

Oximeter   A device worn on the finger or earlobe that can measure levels of oxygen in the blood painlessly. It is one of the measurements made during a sleep study to assess the severity of OSA.

Oxygen   An odorless, colorless gas that makes up 21 percent of the atmosphere of the Earth. Oxygen is necessary for most forms of life and is absorbed through the lungs into the blood.

Palate   The roof of the mouth made up of a hard bony part and a soft muscular part. The soft part has an extension called the *uvula* and is important for speech production, swallowing, and vibration, producing the noise of snoring.

Pharynx   A technical term for the upper part of the throat at the base or back of the tongue.

Polysomnography   A technical term for a *sleep study* that involves recording brain waves for assessing the quality of sleep, airflow at the nose and mouth as well as efforts made to breathe, electrocardiogram, and other parameters including blood oxygen levels, in order to determine the nature and severity of a sleep-related breathing problem. The study is painless and noninvasive.

Pulmonary   A term that relates to the lungs or the artery that takes blood from the right side of the heart to the lungs.

Pulmonary hypertension   A term a doctor may use when talking about high blood pressure in the pulmonary artery. This occurs when oxygen levels in the alveoli in the lungs are low because of lung disease or because fresh air does not get into the lungs due to a blockage in the oropharynx caused by OSA.

Retina   The structure inside the eye that receives light and begins its processing for the brain.

Rhinitis   The technical term used for a runny or congested nose. *Rhino* refers to the "nose" and *itis* means "inflammation or swelling."

Snoring   The noise produced by vibration of the soft palate and uvula.

Tonsils   Structures located on both sides of the oropharynx that may cause narrowing of the airway if enlarged.

Trachea   The main airway that divides into large bronchial tubes going to each lung.

Turbinates   Tubular structures that project into the nasal chambers and increase the surface area of the walls inside the nose. A mucous membrane that is rich in blood vessels covers these turbinates. The turbinates may swell and cause nasal obstruction.

Uvula   A cone-shaped projection hanging down from the soft palate in the oropharynx. The uvula may become swollen and enlarged in people who snore.

Resources

American Sleep Disorders Association
http://www.asda.org

SleepNet
http://www.sleepnet.com

Sleep Apnea

Mayo Health Oasis
http://www.mayohealth.org/mayo/9803/htm/apnea.htm

National Institutes of Health
http://www.ninds.nih.gov/healinfo/disorder/sleep/sleep.htm

Sleep Foundation
http://www.sleepfoundation.org/publications/sleepap.htm

Snoring

Mayo Health Oasis
http://www.mayohealth.org/mayo/9507/htm/snoring.htm

University of Washington
http://weber.u.washington.edu/~Eotoweb/sleepapnea.html

ORGANIZATIONS

American Academy of Neurology
1080 Montreal Avenue
St. Paul, MN 55116
Telephone: 612-695-1940

American College of Chest Physicians
3300 Dundee Road
Northbrook, IL 60062-2348
Telephone: 847-498-1400
Fax: 847-498-5460

American Dietetic Association
Toll free telephone: 800-366-1655

American Sleep Apnea Association
2025 Pennsylvania Avenue NW
Suite 905
Washington, DC 20006
Telephone: 202-293-3650
Fax: 202-293-3656

American Sleep Disorders Association
6301 Bandel Road
Suite 101
Rochester, MN 55901
Telephone: 507-287-6006
Fax: 507-287-6008

American Thoracic Society
1740 Broadway
New York, NY 10019
Telephone: 212-315-8700

Association of Polysomnographic Technologists
8310 Nieman Road
Lenexa, KS 66214
Telephone: 913-541-1991

National Sleep Foundation
729 Fifteenth Street, NW
Fourth Floor
Washington, DC 20005

Sleep Research Society
1610 14th Street Northwest
Suite 300
Rochester, MN 55901
Telephone: 507-287-6006
Fax: 507-287-6008

JOURNALS

Journal of Sleep Research
(Journal Subscriptions)
PO Box 88
Oxford OX2 0NE
United Kingdom

Sleep
1610 14th Street Northwest
Suite 304
Rochester, MN 55901
Telephone: 507-529-0804
Fax: 507-287-6008

Index